Audiology Clinical Protocols

Prepared by the staff of the
University of Minnesota Hospital Audiology Clinic

Robert H. Margolis, Director
John H. Anderson
Eric M. Fournier
Barbara Friedman
Judith E. Hirsch
Lisa L. Hunter
Catherine Jons
Jennifer L. Schmitz
Sharon L. Smith

Allyn and Bacon
Boston · London · Toronto · Sydney · Tokyo · Singapore

ISBN 0-205-26824-2

Printed in the United States of America

10 9 8 7 6 5 4 3 2 1   02 01 00 99 98 97

Table of Contents

Foreword

In 1988, soon after I joined the faculty as Director of Audiology in the University of Minnesota Department of Otolaryngology, I visited the audiology clinic at Good Samaritan Hospital in Portland, Oregon, then directed by Dr. David Lilly. The idea for this protocol book originated with that visit. Dr. Lilly had prepared written protocols for some of the procedures performed in his clinic to guide other clinicians. I thought that a written protocol for each of the services provided by our clinic would be an excellent method for insuring quality control by requiring periodic review and updating of procedures.

Since then, a written protocol has been developed for each service provided by the University of Minnesota Hospital Audiology Clinic. Protocols were assigned to staff members who prepared a first draft for discussion, after which the protocol was revised and approved by consensus. It took about a year and a half to develop the first versions of each of the original protocols. Once this was completed, we began again to review and revise each protocol. One protocol is scheduled for discussion at each of our biweekly staff meetings. Most of the protocols have been revised three or four times since the original version was approved. A few protocols, such as Facial Nerve Electroneurography and Central Auditory Processing Evaluation were added after the first round of protocols was developed.

This process has been beneficial in ways that we did not anticipate. Most importantly, it provided a mechanism by which staff could discuss, justify, and sometimes argue about what we do. Procedures that could not be justified were dropped. Protocols were streamlined to obtain the important information as efficiently as possible. As new methods emerged, protocols were revised or replaced. The protocols are read by all of the students and clinical fellows that participate in the activities in the Clinic, and they have proven to have significant educational value. In fact, the positive response of many of our students was a factor in the decision to publish this book.

The staff of the University of Minnesota Hospital wish to thank Dr. Lilly for the idea for this book, to Sharon Smith for the many hours required to compile the individual protocols into a single document, and to Denise Hove for the final copy editing and formatting. We are grateful to the Lions 5M Hearing Foundation for their support of the University of Minnesota Lions International Hearing Center, without whose support the Clinic could not provide many of the services described in this book.

Robert H. Margolis, Ph.D.
Professor, Department of Otolaryngology
Director of Audiology
September, 1996

Introduction to Protocols

A few underlying assumptions guided the development of this book and should be considered in utilizing these protocols. First, in developing and evaluating clinical procedures our respect for our patients must be the highest priority. That respect requires that inclusion of a procedure in a protocol must be justified in terms of benefit to the patient. The clinician needs to consider whether the time, money, and in some cases, discomfort associated with a procedure is offset by benefit to the patient. In some cases, the benefit cannot be determined until the procedure has been performed. Nonetheless, there must sufficient *potential* benefit to warrant the procedure. Second, these protocols were developed with the full understanding that clinical procedures must be tailored to the needs of the patient. No protocol should be rigidly administered. Procedures are modified, replaced, or eliminated based on clinical judgement of the needs of the patient. This book is not intended as a strict formula for clinical practice. Third, protocols were written so that none were specific to a particular piece of equipment. Equipment-specific information has been included in appendices where the information was judged to be useful. Fourth, in preparing these protocols, a delicate balance was sought between detailed "cookbook" descriptions and more general clinical guidelines. It is not expected that an inexperienced clinician can read these protocols and perform these services. Some clinical procedures, such as Tympanic Electrocochleography and Pediatric Central Auditory Processing Evaluation, require skills and experiences that many audiologists do not possess. This book does not replace the need for proper training and supervision.

Each Protocol is organized into the following sections:

Target Population
Equipment Required
Methods
Report Format
Billing
References
Appendices

The **Target Population** is the group of patients that are expected to benefit from the procedure. In some cases, a protocol may be appropriate for other patients as well.

Equipment Required lists the minimum physical resources that are required to administer the protocol. The equipment listed in each protocol, to some extent, reflects the preferences of the clinicians that developed this manual. Other equipment may be appropriate. This book does not attempt to evaluate audiometric equipment or provide guidance for the selection of clinic instrumentation nor does it describe calibration procedures. The assumption is made that equipment used for the administration of the procedures described in this book is appropriate, in good repair, and properly calibrated.

The **Methods** describe the procedures, usually, but not always, in the order that they are administered. The Methods should be regarded as tools that are used to obtain specific types of information. If other tools are available for achieving the goal, such as case history or previous test results, then the methods should be modified accordingly.

Report Format indicates the manner with which the results are reported and the locations in which reports are archived. Most reports are filed in the hospital chart; some are filed in the hearing aid chart that is separate from hospital medical records. For most protocols a sample report is provided. Reporting requirements differ widely at different centers. The reporting procedures described in this manual should not be regarded as universally appropriate.

Billing Information is based on an assessment of the effort and resources required for each protocol. Appropriate Physicians' Current Procedural Terminology (CPT codes) that are used for billing are indicated. The descriptors used to identify procedures in the protocols do not always correspond exactly to the terms used in the designation of CPT codes. However, the CPT codes indicated are those used to bill for the services described in each protocol. No dollar figures are given.

References are provided to indicate sources of information that may help understand the design of the protocol.

Appendices include a variety of forms, sample reports, and additional information that may be useful in understanding the details of a procedure.

A Note on Infection Control

Like other health care providers, audiologists are expected to take appropriate and effective measures to prevent transmission of disease from patient to patient, from patient to clinician, and from clinician to patient. This requires an infection control regimen that is integrated into the day-to-day operation of the clinic. Several regulatory agencies, including the Joint Commission for the Accreditation of Healthcare Organizations (JCAHO), the Environmental Protection Agency (EPA), the Occupational Safety and Health Administration (OSHA), the Food and Drug Administration (FDA), as well as state and local agencies, have developed guidelines and regulations for infection control procedures and products. All healthcare providers should be knowledgeable about infection control requirements for their workplace.

Because the delivery of audiology services requires contact between the patient and clinician and between the patient and equipment that will eventually contact others, audiologists must be knowledgeable about the potential for disease transmission and effective preventive measures. Depending on the nature of the patient contact, audiometric equipment may require simple cleaning, antimicrobial disinfection, or sterilization. Particular care must be taken when the potential for contact with body fluids exists. Supra-aural earphones, insert earphones, ear canal probe tips (used for acoustic immittance and otoacoustic emissions testing), otoscope specula, probe tubes, stock earmolds, and illuminated probes (for placing otoblocks) are obvious potential hazards for infectious transmission. Less obvious are toys for play audiometry, work surfaces, furniture, and waiting room materials (such as magazines and toys). Virtually everything in the clinic should be included in an organized regimen of infection control. Hospital-based clinics can obtain assistance and advice from the infection control department in the hospital, which maintains and administers hospital-wide policies and procedures.

A complete description of infection control procedures for audiology clinics is not within the scope of this book. The reader is referred to the excellent recent reviews of the topic listed below.

REFERENCES ON INFECTION CONTROL

Ballachanda, B. B. (1995). *The Human Ear Canal.* San Diego: Singular Publishing Group, Inc. (see Appendix B)

Ballachanda, B. B., Roeser, R. J., & Kemp, R. J. (1996). Control and prevention of disease transmission in audiology practice. *American Journal of Audiology* , *5,* 74-82.

Kemp, R.J., Roeser, R.J., Pearson, D.W., & Ballachanda, B.B. (1996). *Infection Control for the Professions of Audiology and Speech-Language Pathology.* Olathe, KS: Iles Publications.

Section I **Auditory Evaluation**

Protocol 1 **Basic Hearing Evaluation**

Target Population:
All patients who can be tested by behavioral audiometry a) have concerns about their hearing, b) require hearing evaluation to determine hearing aid candidacy, or c) are referred for hearing evaluation as part of a medical evaluation.

Rationale:
The first step in the auditory assessment and aural rehabilitation process of a hearing-impaired patient is to obtain test results that will allow a complete characterization of the extent and nature of the hearing impairment. The basic evaluation is typically conducted on the first visit. Abbreviated evaluations may be performed on subsequent visits.

Equipment Required:
Otoscope
Clinical audiometer with pure tone and recorded speech capabilities, supra-aural (TDH-50) and insert (ER-3A) earphones
Aural acoustic immittance system

Methods:
1.   History. The patient will fill out an Adult Case History Form (Appendix A) prior to testing. The form covers hearing problems, ear surgery, medications, tinnitus, dizziness, noise exposure and hearing aid history. If any questions are answered to the affirmative, further questioning may be appropriate.

2.   Visual Inspection. The outer ear will be inspected for any gross abnormalities that would prevent testing or warrant consultation with a physician. If drainage or blood is seen, the tester will wear protective gloves and place covers over the earphones. If supra-aural earphones will be used, the outer ear will be evaluated for its ability to support TDH-50 earphones. When there is concern for its ability to do so, insert earphones will be used. The ear canals will be inspected otoscopically to rule out ear canal occlusion. If the ear canals are occluded to the extent that hearing test results may be affected, follow the steps outlined in Protocol 3   Cerumen Removal. When blood or effusion is observed in either ear canal, a physician will be consulted before proceeding with the evaluation.

3.   Pure-Tone Threshold Audiometry. The procedure for determining threshold will be that described in ANSI S3.21 (1978) Procedure for Manual Pure-Tone Threshold Audiometry.
    a.   Pure-tone thresholds for air-conduction stimuli will be obtained for standard octave audiometric frequencies from 250 through 8000 Hz using either supra-aural or insert earphones. Insert earphones will be used when: there is concern regarding canal collapse, bilateral conductive hearing loss is suspected, or head shape or size is too small or too large to accommodate use of supra-aural earphones. Inter-octave

frequencies will be tested when a difference of ≥ 20 dB occurs in thresholds of two adjacent octave frequencies. In certain cases other frequencies must be tested. The calculation of hearing handicap by Workman's Compensation and AAO methods requires a threshold at 3000 Hz. When hearing aids may be ordered, thresholds are measured at 1500 and 3000 Hz. In cases of possible ototoxicity, 3000 and 6000-Hz thresholds are also measured.

b.   Bone-conduction thresholds will be obtained at any octave audiometric frequency, excluding 8000 Hz, at which the air-conduction threshold is ≥ 15 dB HL or when middle ear disease is suspected. Contralateral masking will be used in air-conduction and bone-conduction testing when appropriate.

4.   <u>Word-Recognition Test</u>. A word-recognition test will be administered monaurally to each ear with recorded Northwestern University NU-6 materials. A ten word list can be used if hearing is within normal limits and no auditory symptoms exist, or if the loss is purely conductive and a score of 100% was obtained on the previous evaluation. If one or more errors occurs on the first ten items or a sensorineural hearing loss exists, at least 25 test items will be presented. Test materials will be presented at 40 dB above the three frequency pure tone average provided this level is at least 10 dB above all thresholds from 500-3000 Hz. If the 40-dB level does not achieve audibility through 3000 Hz, the presentation level is increased as appropriate, provided tolerance and audiometric limits will allow. In certain cases a lower sensation level may be required in order to obtain the maximum word recognition score. If scores are inconsistent with the pure-tone results or previous results or symptoms suggest retrocochlear pathology, the test will be repeated at one or more higher sensation levels. The higher level will be 90 dB HL or higher (when tolerance and audiometer limits allow) and at least 20-dB above the lower presentation level in order to determine if performance rollover exists. A rollover index of 0.45 or greater is considered significant (see Appendix B for Calculation Of The Rollover Index). Contralateral masking using speech noise will be used in word-recognition testing when appropriate.

5.   <u>Tympanometry</u>. Tympanograms for each ear will be obtained with a 226-Hz probe frequency. Air pressure will be swept in the positive-to-negative direction at a rate of 250 daPa/s. (Appendix C describes the fail criteria for tympanometric variables.) If middle ear pathology is suspected, or an air-bone gap of ≥ 10 dB HL at two or more frequencies exists in the presence of peaked 226-Hz tympanograms, estimates of middle-ear resonance in both ears will be obtained using multifrequency tympanometry. The frequency range tested will be 500-2000 Hz (1/6 octave steps) with a pressure range of +500 to -400 daPa (a narrower pressure range of +200 to -300 daPa can be used if problems exist maintaining the probe seal). The sweep pressure method will be used if a high-impedance pathology is suspected. The sweep frequency method will be used if a low-impedance pathology is suspected. An estimate of the middle-ear resonant frequency is the probe frequency at which the minimum of the susceptance (B) tympanogram notch reaches the positive tail of the tympanogram. Tympanometric patterns will also be evaluated to determine consistency with the Vanhuyse model. (Refer to Appendix D for normal resonant frequency ranges for children and adults.)

6.   <u>Acoustic-Reflex Test</u>. For each ear in patients with normal hearing or symmetrical sensorineural hearing loss and no suspicion of retrocochlear lesion, threshold of the ipsilateral acoustic reflex will be determined. Contralateral acoustic reflexes may be obtained when the interpretation of ipsilateral reflex is hindered by artifact, thresholds are inconsistent with the

pure tone audiogram, or retrocochlear or brainstem pathologies are suspected. A 1000-Hz eliciting stimulus with a probe frequency of 226 Hz will be used. Thresholds will be determined by one descending series of stimuli with a step size of 5 dB. When thresholds are inconsistent with the pure tone audiogram or previous results suggest retrocochlear pathology, additional acoustic reflex threshold test frequencies, e.g. 500 and 2000 Hz, and acoustic reflex decay may be measured. Appendix E presents the normal range and upper limits of acoustic reflexes for various degree and types of hearing losses.

7.   Speech Recognition Thresholds. SRTs may be obtained to confirm pure tone results or when pseudohypacusis is suspected. When SRTs are obtained to confirm pure tone results, a descending method will be used, by presenting spondees (monitored live voice) at suprathreshold levels and then decreasing the level of presentation in 5 dB steps until one word is missed. Three words are presented at that level. SRT is defined at the lowest level where 2 of 3 words are repeated correctly. In cases of non-English speaking patients, informal procedures for speech recognition utilizing an interpreter may be employed. SRTs that differ from pure tone averages by more than 10-15 dB, in the absence of explanations such as the slope of the audiogram or poor word recognition will be considered suggestive of pseudohypacusis.

8.   Pseudohypacusis Hearing Loss.
        a.   The Stenger and/or Speech Stenger (Martin, 1994) will be performed on all patients presenting a unilateral or an asymmetrical (≥ 20 dB inter-aural difference) hearing loss.
        b.   If acoustic-reflex thresholds are less than 25 dB above pure tone thresholds, pseudohypacusis should be considered.
        c.   Speech recognition thresholds (SRT) will be obtained, using an ascending method, with patients suspected of pseudohypacusis.

9.   Tuning Fork Tests. If questions exist regarding the presence of a conductive component, tuning fork tests will be performed as described in Appendix F.

10.   Referral for an Otologic Examination will be made if the patient has one or more of the following:
        a.   a conductive loss of ≥ 10 dB HL at two or more octave frequencies
        b.   a fluctuating or sudden onset sensorineural hearing loss
        c.   an asymmetric sensorineural hearing loss
        d.   dizziness
        e.   tinnitus not explained by noise induced hearing loss
        f.   otalgia or otorrhea
        g.   aural fullness
        h.   other symptoms that may be associated with otologic disease
        i.   a recommendation for a hearing aid

11.   Postcards. For patients requiring annual or semi-annual follow-up appointments, postcards will be filled out by the patients and filed by the audiologist and placed in the card file to be mailed to the patient as a reminder for their follow-up appointments.

Report Format:
Test results will be saved on the "Patient Audio" and "Patient Tymps" file servers and recorded on the Audiologic Record Form (see Appendix G). Appropriate comments will be entered on the bottom of the form.

Billing:
Bill Audiogram, either "Audiogram-Air & Bone" (CPT 92553) or "Audiogram-Air" (CPT 92552); 1 unit per ear.
Bill Speech Audiometry (CPT 92556); 1 unit for each 25-word list; 1 unit for 2 10-word lists; 1 unit for SRT testing for both ears (CPT 92555).
Bill Tympanometry (CPT 92567); 1 unit per ear, 1 additional unit per ear if multifrequency testing is done.
Bill Acoustic Reflexes (CPT 92568) and Decay (CPT 92569); 1 unit per threshold; 1 unit per decay test.
Bill Stenger (CPT 92565); 1 unit per frequency tested

References:

American National Standards Institute. (1978). *American National Standards Method for Manual Pure-Tone Threshold Audiometry.* (ANSI S3.21-1978). New York.

Bess, F. H. (1983). Clinical assessment of speech recognition. In D. F. Konkle and W. F. Rintelmann (Eds.), *Principles of Speech Audiometry* (pp. 127-202). New York: Prentice Hall.

Dirks, D. D., Kamm, C., Bower, D., & Betsworth, A. (1977). Use of performance-Intensity functions for diagnosis. *Journal of Speech and Hearing Disorders, 42,* 408-415.

Hunter, L. L., & Margolis, R. H. (1992). Multifrequency tympanometry: Current clinical application. *American Journal of Audiology, 4,* 33-43.

Margolis, R. H., & Goycoolea, H. (1993). Multifrequency tympanometry in normal adults. *Ear and Hearing, 14,* 408-413.

Margolis, R. H., & Shanks, J. E. (1991). Tympanometry: Basic principles and clinical applications. In W. F. Rintelmann (Ed.), *Hearing Assessment* (pp. 179-247, 2nd Ed.). Austin, Texas: Pro-Ed.

Martin, F. N. (1994). Pseudohypacusis. In J. Katz (Ed.), *Handbook of Clinical Audiology* (pp. 553-567, 4th. Ed.). Baltimore, MD: Williams and Wilkins.

Northern, J. L., & Gabbard, S. A. (1994). The acoustic reflex. In J. Katz (Ed.), *Handbook of Clinical Audiology* (pp. 300-316, 4th Ed.). Baltimore, MD: Williams and Wilkins.

Olsen, W. O., & Matkin, N. D. (1991). Speech audiometry. In W.F. Rintelmann (Ed.), *Hearing Assessment* (pp. 39-140, 2nd Ed.). Austin, TX: Pro-Ed.

Popelka, G. R. (Ed.) (1981). *Hearing Assessment With the Acoustic Reflex.* New York: Grune and Stratton.

Wilson, R. H., & Margolis, R. H. (1991). Acoustic-Reflex Measurements. In W.F. Rintelmann (Ed.), *Hearing Assessment* (pp. 247-319, 2nd Ed.). Austin, Texas: Pro-Ed.

Protocol 1 Appendix

ADULT HISTORY

DATE		
	PATIENT INDENtIFICATION PLATE	
NAME	AGE	OCCUPATION
WHO REFERRED YOU TO THE AUDIOLOGY CLINIC?		

WHAT CONCERNS YOU MOST?
☐ HEARING LOSS ☐ DIZZINESS ☐ EAR NOISES ☐ OTHER (specify)

1. IF YOU THINK YOU HAVE A HEARING PROBLEM, PLEASE ANSWER THE FOLLOWING,
   IF NOT, GO TO NO. 2

   a. Do you have a problem in the following situations? (please check)

      ☐ While listening to another person at a distance of 6 feet   ☐ In groups and noisy places

      ☐ At work

      ☐ While using the telephone
         ☐ Left ear   ☐ Right ear   ☐ At home
         ☐ No preference

      ☐ In social/recreational situations

   b. From which ear do you hear better?   ☐ Left   ☐ Right   ☐ Both same

   c. What do you think caused your hearing loss?   _____

   d. Did your hearing loss come on: ☐ Suddenly   ☐ Gradually

   e. When did you first notice loss?   _____

   f. Has it gotten worse over time?   ☐ Yes   ☐ No

   g. Does it fluctuate from time to time?   ☐ Yes   ☐ No

   h. Does anyone in your family have a hearing problem?   ☐ Yes   ☐ No
      Who?   _____

2. HAVE YOU EVER HAD EAR SURGERY?   ☐ Yes   ☐ No

3. DO YOU PRESENTLY HAVE "TUBES" IN YOUR EARS?   ☐ Yes   ☐ No   ☐ Don't know

4. DO YOU TAKE ANY MEDICINES REGULARLY?   ☐ Yes   ☐ No

5. ARE YOU BOTHERED BY NOISES IN YOUR EARS/HEAD?   ☐ Yes   ☐ No | IF "YES", ☐ Right   ☐ Left   ☐ Both

6. ARE YOU EVER DIZZY?   ☐ Yes   ☐ No | IF "YES", DESCRIBE

7. HAVE YOU EVER BEEN EXPOSED TO LOUD NOISES FOR ANY LENGTH OF TIME?   ☐ Yes   ☐ No | IF "YES", HOW LONG?

8. HAVE YOU EVER USED A HEARING AID IN THE PAST?   ☐ Yes   ☐ No

9. IF YOU ARE USING A HEARING AID NOW, PLEASE ANSWER THE FOLLOWING, IF YOU ARE
   NOT USING AN AID, GO ON TO NO. 10.

   a. Which ear is aided?   ☐ Left   ☐ Right   ☐ Both

   b. How long have you used an aid?

   c. How long have you had your present aid?   _____

   d. Are you satisfied with the aid?   ☐ Yes   ☐ No

10. WHAT DO YOU WANT TO LEARN FROM YOUR VISIT TODAY?

CALCULATION OF ROLLOVER INDEX

$$\text{Rollover Index} = \frac{\text{PB max} - \text{PB min}}{\text{PB max}}$$

A rollover index value ≥ 0.45 is considered a positive result for retrocochlear pathology.

Source: Dirks, D. D., Kamm, C., Bower, D., & Betsworth, A. (1977). Use of performance-intensity functions for diagnosis. *Journal of Speech and Hearing Disorders, 42*, 408-415.

FAIL CRITERIA FOR TYMPANOMETRIC VARIABLES

	STATIC ADMITTANCE[1]	TYMPANOMETRIC WIDTH[2]	EQUIVALENT VOLUME[3]
INFANTS	< 0.02 mmho	> 200 daPa	> 1.0 cm^3
CHILDREN[4]	< 0.20 mmho	> 150 daPa	> 1.0 cm^3
ADULTS	< 0.30 mmho	> 110 daPa	> 1.5 cm^3

[1] STATIC ADMITTANCE = Peak Admittance - Admittance at 200 dapa

[2] TYMPANOMETRIC WIDTH is the pressure interval defined by the intersection of a horizontal line at 0.5 peak admittance with the tympanogram

[3] EQUIVALENT VOLUME is the admittance magnitude at 200 dapa

[4] These norms are based on 3 - 6 year old children

Source: Hunter, L. L., & Margolis, R. H. (1992). Multifrequency tympanometry: Current clinical application. *American Journal of Audiology, 4*, 33-43.

RESONANT FREQUENCY NORMATIVE DATA

NORMAL (90%) RANGES FOR ADULTS

Sweep Pressure
Susceptance +200   630-1400 Hz

Sweep Frequency
Susceptance +200   800-2000 Hz

Source: Margolis, R. H., & Goycoolea, H. (1993). Multifrequency tympanometry in normal adults. *Ear and Hearing, 14*, 408-413.

NORMAL (90%) RANGES FOR CHILDREN AGE 3-10 YEARS

Sweep Pressure
Susceptance +200   755-1425

Sweep Frequency
Susceptance +200   850-1525

Source: Hunter, L. L., & Margolis, R. H. (1992). Multifrequency tympanometry: Current clinical application. *American Journal of Audiology, 4*, 33-43.

ACOUSTIC REFLEX THRESHOLDS

Acoustic Reflexes: Normal Hearing

Auditory Threshold	Acoustic Reflex Threshold
< 40 dB HL	80-90 dB HL
< 40 dB HL	95 dB HL for 250 through 2000-Hz stimuli

Acoustic Reflexes: Conductive Hearing Loss
Ipsilateral and contralateral acoustic reflexes are absent in the presence of even a mild conductive hearing loss.

Acoustic Reflexes: Cochlear Hearing Loss

Auditory Threshold	Acoustic Reflex Threshold
< 40 dB HL	80-90 dB HL
40 to 60 dB HL	Linear increase in acoustic reflex thresholds
> 60 dB HL	15% have absent acoustic reflexes
> 70 dB HL	More likely to have absent acoustic reflexes

Acoustic Reflexes: Eighth Nerve Lesion

Auditory Threshold	Acoustic Reflex Threshold
0 dB HL	30% have absent acoustic reflexes
30 dB HL	70% have absent acoustic reflexes
> 40 db HL	80 to 100% have absent acoustic reflexes

Sources:
Wilson, R. H., & Margolis, R. H. (1991). Acoustic-reflex measurements. In W.F. Rintelmann (Ed.), *Hearing Assessment* (pp. 247-319, 2nd Ed.). Austin, Texas: Pro-Ed.

Northern, J. L., & Gabbard, S. A. (1994). The acoustic reflex. In J. Katz (Ed.), *Handbook of Clinical Audiology* (pp. 300-316, 4th Ed.). Baltimore, MD: Williams and Wilkins.

PROCEDURES FOR AUDIOMETRIC TUNING FORK TESTS

Tuning fork tests are performed with the bone vibrator by holding the spring headband attachment to the vibrator. For uniformity of stimulus levels, it is best not to hold the plastic vibrator case directly. The test frequency should be below 1 kHz, typically 500 Hz. The stimulus level should be 10-20 dB above the air conduction threshold of the poorer ear.

The wording of questions is very important. Care should be taken not to ask leading questions that bias the patient's responses. "Is it louder in the right ear?" is a leading question. "In which ear is it louder" is a more proper form of the question.

Weber Test

The Weber test is performed by holding the vibrator firmly to the midline of the forehead. The patient is asked, "Do you hear the tone?" If the answer is yes, ask "Where do you hear it?" If the answer is indefinite, ask "Is it louder in one ear than the other?"

Interpretation. The Weber lateralizes to 1) the better cochlea; 2) the ear with the greater conductive loss; 3) the ear with the leading phase response; 4) the ear with the better middle ear transmission of bone conducted signals. These processes account for lateralization to the better ear of a patient with sensorineural hearing loss, the poorer ear of a patient with conductive loss, the poorer ear of the patient with ossicular fixation, and the fluid-filled ear, respectively. The test result is reported by indicating the ear to which the Weber lateralized along with the frequency and level of the stimulus.

Bing Test

The Bing test is performed by placing the vibrator on the midline of the forehead and occluding the ear canal by pressing firmly on the tragus. The patient is instructed to "Tell me if the tone gets louder, softer, or stays the same when I push in." If the sound lateralizes to the midline or opposite ear, another appropriate question is "Where do you hear it?" after the ear canal is occluded.

Interpretation. The occlusion of the ear canal produces an occlusion effect which results in a lateralized image and enhanced loudness in the occluded ear. Because the test was originally intended to test for sensorineural hearing loss, a negative result (no occlusion effect) implies conductive loss. The result is reported as negative or positive for each ear along with the frequency and level of the stimulus.

Rinne Test

The Rinne test is performed by placing the vibrator on the mastoid process and then in front of the external auditory meatus. It should be pushed firmly to the mastoid and placed as close to the ear canal entrance as possible without touching the pinna with the circular contact surface facing the ear canal. The patient is asked "Is it louder here or here?" as the vibrator is moved from one position to the other.

Interpretation. Like the Bing test, the Rinne test was originally used as a test for sensorineural hearing loss. Thus a negative Rinne (louder by bone conduction) indicates a conductive loss. The Rinne will be negative if the air-bone gap is greater than approximately 15 dB. A false negative Rinne occurs when the bone conducted stimulus is heard in a better hearing contralateral ear. It is advisable to ask the patient in which ear the bone conduction stimulus is heard when testing each ear with the Rinne test.

AUDIOLOGY RECORD EXAMPLE

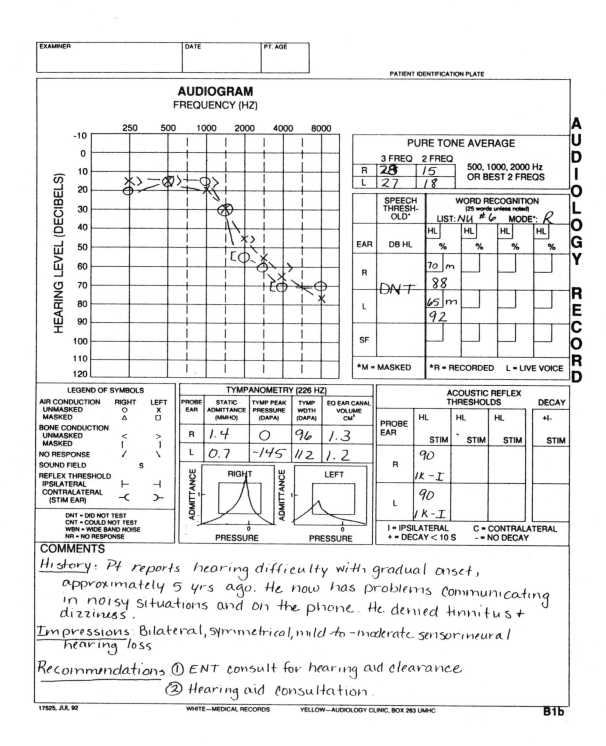

EXAMINER	DATE	PT. AGE

PATIENT IDENTIFICATION PLATE

AUDIOGRAM
FREQUENCY (HZ)

HEARING LEVEL (DECIBELS)

PURE TONE AVERAGE

	3 FREQ	2 FREQ	500, 1000, 2000 Hz OR BEST 2 FREQS
R	28	15	
L	27	18	

	SPEECH THRESH-OLD*	WORD RECOGNITION (25 words unless noted) LIST: NU #6 MODE*: R

EAR	DB HL	HL %	HL %	HL %	HL %
R	DNT	70 m 88			
L		65 m 92			
SF					

*M = MASKED   *R = RECORDED   L = LIVE VOICE

LEGEND OF SYMBOLS

AIR CONDUCTION	RIGHT	LEFT
UNMASKED	O	X
MASKED	Δ	☐
BONE CONDUCTION		
UNMASKED	<	>
MASKED	[	]
NO RESPONSE	/	\
SOUND FIELD	S	
REFLEX THRESHOLD		
IPSILATERAL	⊢	⊣
CONTRALATERAL (STIM EAR)	⊰	⊱

DNT - DID NOT TEST
CNT - COULD NOT TEST
WBN - WIDE BAND NOISE
NR - NO RESPONSE

TYMPANOMETRY (226 HZ)

PROBE EAR	STATIC ADMITTANCE (MMHO)	TYMP PEAK PRESSURE (DAPA)	TYMP WDTH (DAPA)	EQ EAR CANAL VOLUME CM³
R	1.4	0	96	1.3
L	0.7	-145	112	1.2

RIGHT   LEFT

ADMITTANCE   ADMITTANCE

PRESSURE   PRESSURE

ACOUSTIC REFLEX THRESHOLDS   **DECAY**

PROBE EAR	HL STIM	HL STIM	HL STIM	+/- STIM
R	90 1k - I			
L	90 1k - I			

I = IPSILATERAL   C = CONTRALATERAL
+ = DECAY < 10 S   - = NO DECAY

COMMENTS

History: Pt reports hearing difficulty with gradual onset, approximately 5 yrs ago. He now has problems communicating in noisy situations and on the phone. He denied tinnitus + dizziness.

Impressions: Bilateral, symmetrical, mild to-moderate sensorineural hearing loss

Recommendations ① ENT consult for hearing aid clearance
                ② Hearing aid consultation.

AUDIOLOGY RECORD

Protocol 2 **Audiometric Screening**

Target Population:
Any patient who can be tested by behavioral audiometric screening methods and has been referred for a quick and inexpensive hearing procedure.

Rationale:
For certain groups of patients, it is desirable to perform a quick protocol to rule out probable hearing impairment and middle ear dysfunction.

Equipment Required:
Otoscope
Screening audiometer or portable audiometer
Tympanometer

Methods:
1.   <u>Case History</u>. The patient will be questioned regarding history of otalgia, otorrhea, tinnitus, and dizziness. Any recent occurrence of any of the above will be recorded under Comments on the Audiometric Screening Report and a recommendation will be made for medical follow-up.

2.   <u>Visual Examination</u>. The head and neck will be examined for developmental abnormalities. The ear canals will be inspected otoscopically for abnormalities such as blood, effusion, occlusion, inflammation, excessive cerumen, or foreign material. The eardrums will be inspected otoscopically for abnormalities such as abnormal color, bulging eardrum, fluid line, bubbles, perforation, or retraction. Any defect of the head or neck, or abnormal otoscopic finding will be reported as a fail.

3.   <u>Pure-Tone Audiometric Screen</u>. Audiometric screening will be performed in accordance with the Guidelines for Identification Audiometry (Asha, 1985). Pure-tone screening will be administered to each ear at four frequencies (500, 1000, 2000, and 4000 Hz) at 20 dB HL. In situations where background noise is present, a higher intensity screening level may be required. If so, the examiner should do a psychophysical threshold check and use a screening level 5 dB re: the examiner's threshold. The examiner's thresholds should be recorded on the Audiometric Screening Report and it should be noted under the audiogram that the screening levels were adjusted due to ambient noise. Absence of a response to any of the eight stimuli will be reported as a fail.

4.   <u>Tympanometric Screen</u>. Tympanograms will be obtained from each ear with a 226-Hz probe frequency. The following quantities, which are described in Appendix A, will be obtained from the tympanograms:

  a.   Equivalent ear-canal volume
  b.   Peak compensated static acoustic admittance
  c.   Tympanometric width

A flat tympanogram will be reported as a fail and the equivalent volume will be mentioned under Comments on the Audiometric Screen Report. All patients with flat tympanograms, abnormally low static admittance, or abnormally wide tympanometric width will be referred for medical follow-up. Abnormally high static admittance, abnormally narrow tympanometric width, and abnormal tympanometric peak pressure are not cause for failing the screen. Fail criteria for tympanometric variables are given in Appendix B.

Report Format:
Results will be reported on the Audiometric Screen Report (Appendix A).

If a patient fails the Audiometric Screening, the audiologist should report to the referring physician, explain the results, and request a full evaluation.

Billing:
Bill Audiometric Screening (CPT 92551).

References:
American Speech-Language-Hearing Association. (1985, May). Guidelines for identification audiometry. *Asha, 27,* 49-52.

American Speech-Language-Hearing Association. (1990). Guidelines for screening for hearing impairment and middle ear disorders. *Asha, 32* (Supplement 2), 17-24.

Margolis, R. H., & Heller, J. W. (1987). Screening tympanometry: Criteria for medical referral. *Audiology, 26,* 197-208.

Protocol 2 Appendix

A.   Audiometric Screening Form
B.   Fail Criteria for Tympanometric Variables

AUDIOMETRIC SCREENING

Patient Name: _____   Hospital ID# _____

Date ____-____-____   Audiologist: _____

VISUAL INSPECTION: RIGHT EAR   LEFT EAR

                                _____   _____

PURE TONE SCREEN: _____   dBHL

FREQ (Hz):	500	1000	2000	4000
RIGHT				
LEFT				

TYMPANOMETRY: RIGHT EAR   LEFT EAR

                                _____   _____

+ = PASS
- = FAIL

COMMENTS:

FAIL CRITERIA FOR TYMPANOMETRIC VARIABLES

	STATIC ADMITTANCE[1]	TYMPANOMETRIC WIDTH[2]	EQUIVALENT VOLUME[3]
CHILDREN[4]	< 0.20 mmho	> 150 daPa	> 1.0 cm³
ADULTS	< 0.30 mmho	> 110 daPa	> 1.5 cm³

[1] STATIC ADMITTANCE = Peak Admittance - Admittance at 200 dapa

[2] TYMPANOMETRIC WIDTH is the pressure interval defined by the intersection of a horizontal line at 0.5 peak admittance with the tympanogram

[3] EQUIVALENT VOLUME is the admittance magnitude at 200 dapa

[4] These norms are based on 3 - 6 year old children

Source: Hunter, L. L., & Margolis, R. H. (1992). Multifrequency tympanometry: Current clinical application. *American Journal of Audiology, 4,* 33-43.

Protocol 3 **Cerumen Removal**

Target Population:
1.   Patients who require an earmold impression and have sufficient cerumen to cause an inadequate earmold or those who have enough cerumen that an earmold impression may result in impaction.
2.   Patients who require audiometric testing and have $\geq$ 50% occlusion of the ear canal.
3.   Patients who require testing by tympanic electrocochleography and have sufficient cerumen to impede visualization of the tympanic membrane during electrode placement.
4.   Patients who require real ear acoustical testing and have sufficient cerumen to interfere with proper placement of the probe tube.
5.   Patients who are hearing aid users and have sufficient cerumen to interfere with proper function of the hearing aid.

Rationale:
Excessive cerumen in the ear canal can interfere with obtaining an adequate earmold impression, audiologic testing, and hearing aid function.

Equipment Required:
Headlamp
Surgical microscope
Otoscope specula
Nasal specula
Curettes (2, 3, and 4 mm)
Cotton-tipped swabs
Alligator forceps

Methods:
1.   Otoscopic inspection. An otoscopic inspection is performed to determine the need for cerumen removal. Depending on the amount and depth of cerumen, removal will be performed with a headlamp or with a surgical microscope.

2.   The Cerumen Removal Checklist (see Appendix A) is completed prior to cerumen removal to rule out contraindications.

3.   Contraindications. Under the following circumstances, extreme caution should be exercised when cerumen removal is performed by Audiology personnel. When cerumen removal is particularly difficult due to amount, location, or difficult visualization, the following patients should be referred to ENT.
     a.   Patients with effusion in the ear canal.
     b.   Patients who have had surgical modification of the ear canal wall.
     c.   Patients who are being seen in connection with a legal proceeding.

d.   Patients who are immune suppressed including chemotherapy patients, HIV patients, bone marrow transplant patients, and patients with a white cell count < 4000.

e.   Patients with bleeding disorders, e.g. hemophilia, platelet count < 50,000, or abnormal bleeding time.

f.   Patients who require restraint to accomplish cerumen removal, e.g. young children.

4.   Termination of procedure. Efforts to remove cerumen are terminated if the patient complains of vertigo or severe pain or if bleeding occurs in the ear canal. Under these conditions, the patient is referred to the ENT Clinic.

5.   When the cerumen is located in the lateral portion of the ear canal and is not excessive it will be removed with a headlamp and curette. A nasal speculum or otoscope speculum may be used to assist visualization. Contact between the curette and the skin should be minimized. An alligator forceps can be used to remove loose material.

6.   When the cerumen is excessive and/or located in the medial portion of the ear canal, a surgical microscope will be used. Under direct microscopic visualization, using a speculum to spread the cartilaginous ear canal, cerumen is removed with a curette of appropriate size or alligator forceps.

Report Format:
A chart note is made in the hospital chart indicating that cerumen was removed (specify ear) and describing complications. The Cerumen Removal Checklist is placed in the hearing aid chart or filed in the Audiology Clinic.

Billing:
Bill Wax Removal (CPT 69210); one unit for two ears when the headlamp is used; one unit per ear if the microscope is used. Extra units can be billed for an unusual amount of time.

References:
American Speech-Language-Hearing Association. (1991). External auditory canal examination and cerumen management. *Asha, 35,* 65-66.

Ballachanda B. B., & Peers C. J. (1992). Cerumen management: Instruments and procedures. *Asha, 34,* 43-46.

Protocol 3 Appendix

A.   Cerumen Removal Checklist

CERUMEN REMOVAL CHECKLIST

Patient Name: ___ _____ UMHC# __ _____ **Date** _____

Audiologist: . _____ **Cerumen Removed by:** . _____

Yes   No

Effusion in ear canal.

—   —   Right

—   —   Left

Surgery involving ear canal wall.

—   —   Right

—   —   Left

—   —   Legal proceeding in progress.

—   —   Immune suppressed (chemotherapy, HIV, bone marrow transplant, white cell
                    count <4000).

—   —   Bleeding disorder (e.g. hemophilia, platelet count <50,000, abnormal bleeding
                    time, blood thinning medication).

—   —   Restraint required.

—   —   Recent vertigo or otalgia.

—   —   Recent radiation therapy.

Right Left

—   —   Cerumen removed from

Comments:

Target Population:
Young children, and other individuals, who cannot be tested by conventional behavioral audiometry.

Rationale:
The purpose is to identify hearing impairment for medical management and aural habilitation/ rehabilitation. As much information as possible is needed on the following:

degree of hearing impairment;
type of hearing impairment;
status of middle ear function;
audiometric configuration;
relationship between ears; and,
word-recognition ability.

In order to obtain this information with children, flexibility and multiple procedural alternatives are critical. Also, knowledge on developmental abilities is important in selecting test procedures. The protocol should be designed to obtain the most important information first.

Equipment Required:
Otoscope
Clinical audiometer (pure tone, speech, and soundfield capabilities)
Visual reinforcers for visual reinforcement audiometry (VRA)
Portable audiometer
Tangible reinforcement for operant conditioning audiometer (TROCA)
Variety of toys for conditioned play audiometry
Acoustic immittance system or portable tympanometer
Intercom system
Otoacoustic emissions test equipment

Methods:
1. <u>History</u>. The Pediatric History Form is completed by the caregiver in the waiting room prior to the appointment (Appendix A). If any significant problems are noted on the screening form, the Pediatric Historical Review (Appendix B) should be completed by the audiologist with the caregiver and child in the test suite.

2. <u>Auditory Evaluation</u>. One or more of the following procedures will be used. Exact procedures used are dependent on developmental age and success with other procedures. The goal is to get as complete an audiogram as possible. As much as possible, follow Methods #2 "Pure Tone Threshold Audiometry" outlined in Protocol 1 Basic Hearing Evaluation.
    a. Auditory Brainstem Response (ABR). See Protocol 14 ABR Threshold Evaluation for details. This procedure is not part of Pediatric Hearing Evaluation protocol, but it is

the preferred test for children under 5 months of age, and may be used in conjunction with tests listed below when limited results are obtained or when there is a question of validity. If abnormal results are obtained, behavioral testing should be completed because an abnormal ABR could reflect either an auditory or neurologic problem. See Appendix C for specific instructions.

  b.   Otoacoustic Emissions (OAEs). The purpose of OAEs is either to screen for the presence of significant hearing loss or provide further information about the site of lesion. This procedure should be completed to verify or extend behavioral or ABR results. Either Transient Evoked Otoacoustic Emissions (TEOAEs) or Distortion Product Emissions (DPEs) may be used. If TEOAEs are used refer to Protocol 15 TEOAE Screen. If DPEs are used, the following procedures are recommended. (See Appendix C in Protocol 15 for specific instructions.)

  1.   Select one point per octave over the range 1000-6000 Hz and F2/F1 of 1.2.
  2.   Use equal level primaries of 70 dB SPL.
  3.   If time permits, obtain at least two replications at each point.

If noise level is too high, good recordings at 1000 Hz may be difficult to obtain.

  c.   Behavioral Observation Audiometry (age 0-4 months). Very gross estimates of hearing can be made through observation of any behavioral response (e.g., eye blink, head turn, movement, breathing and voicing changes, etc.) to an acoustic signal. After an initial screen with noisemakers, calibrated stimuli of speech and frequency specific warble tones and narrow-band noises should be utilized. Infants should be seated on the parent's lap with an observer in the room. Use ascending presentations of stimuli with minimal numbers of presentations and long inter-stimulus intervals. This procedure should be used in conjunction with electrophysiological procedures, because it cannot be used to establish auditory threshold.

  d.   Visual Reinforcement Audiometry (VRA) (age 5 months to 3 years). Visual reinforcement of a behavioral response to an auditory signal (speech or frequency-specific stimuli) is used to estimate auditory thresholds. The following are some considerations when implementing this procedure:

  1.   Remove extra visual distractors.
  2.   Position the child on the parent's knees with a visual distractor in front.
  3.   Dim the lights in the examiner's room.
  4.   Use a variety of visual reinforcers.
  5.   Initiate testing in the soundfield. Once completed, try earphone and bone-conduction testing with the same procedure.
  6.   Randomly alternate presentations between speakers to assess threshold and localization ability. If localization is not observed, use one speaker. Initiate testing with long inter-stimulus intervals, 10 dB increments, and an ascending presentation of stimuli (condition at suprathreshold levels when necessary).

Order stimulus presentations in the following manner:

  1.   speech;
  2.   2000-Hz warble-tone (WT) or narrow-band noise (NBN);
  3.   500-Hz WT or NBN; and,
  4.   evaluate remaining audiometric frequencies.

  e.   Conditioned Play Audiometry (ages 2 and older). For new or very young patients, it may be preferable to begin with speech thresholds. The child is conditioned to perform a play-response task when an auditory signal is presented.

  f.   Tangible Reinforcement for Operant Conditioning Audiometry (TROCA) (age 2 and older). The child pushes a response button on a feeder box whenever a sound is perceived. A tangible reinforcer is provided. This procedure should be used if Conditioned Play Audiometry is unsuccessful as it takes much longer to implement.

3.   Speech-Recognition Thresholds (SRT) or Speech-Awareness Thresholds (SAT). Assess SRT or SAT to verify frequency-specific information. This should be done before play audiometry as it gives a quick idea of stimulus levels for conditioning. Better thresholds may be obtained as a speech stimulus than for pure tone stimuli. Stimulus are selected based on the speech and language abilities of the child. The preferred stimuli are spondees, but if they are not successful try pointing to body parts. Specify on the audiogram which measurement was obtained, i.e. SRT or SAT.

4.   Word-Recognition Tests. If sensorineural hearing impairment is suspected, a live voice word-recognition test should be administered to each ear using the NU-CHIPS (for ages 3 & 4 years), the Word Intelligibility by Picture Identification Test (for children ages 4 & 5 years) or PBK word list (for children 3 years of age and older, who have better speech and vocabulary skills). Grosser measures of word recognition, such as identification of selected spondees may be used to obtain some estimate of recognition ability. Test materials will be presented at 40 dB re: pure tone average as specified in Protocol 1 Basic Hearing Evaluation.

Perform steps 5, 6, and 7 first only if it is felt that they will not upset the child and prevent obtaining behavioral results.

5.   Otoscopic Inspection. See Protocol 1 Basic Hearing Evaluation.

6.   Tympanometry. Tympanograms on each ear will be obtained with a 226-Hz probe tone (see Protocol 1 Basic Hearing Evaluation). Air pressure will be changed in the positive-to-negative direction with a rate of 250 daPa/s. For children under four months of age, multifrequency tympanometry should be obtained. When using the portable tympanometer: 2 repetitions that show similar patterns should be obtained to insure replicability.

7.   Acoustic-Reflex Thresholds. If the tympanogram is not flat, and the child is cooperative, follow the method outlined in Protocol 1 Basic Hearing Evaluation.

8.   Speech-Language Screening. If the child is between 0 and 36 months, a speech language screening such as the Early Language Milestone Scale (ELM Scale 2nd Edition, Coplan, 1993) may be performed to evaluate the need to refer for formal speech-language evaluation. Screening may be deleted for children who are obviously not at risk for delay (e.g., no history or current evidence of hearing loss and child observed by audiologist to be speaking clearly in sentences by age 2). If the child has been evaluated by a speech-language pathologist within the past 6 months or is currently receiving speech therapy, screening is also not necessary. Follow procedures as described in the Screening manual to administer and score the test.

9.   Counseling. Thoroughly explain the test results to the child's parents. In the case of a significant hearing loss requiring amplification, the parents may be overwhelmed by the discovery of the loss and the amount of information. See Appendix C for information on special services that should be discussed with parents of hearing-impaired children. If normal results are obtained, recommend follow-up testing when there are suspicions of fluctuating hearing impairment, particularly if any change in behavior is noted.

Report Format:
Results will be recorded on the Audiologic Record Form (Appendix G in Protocol 1). Results should be interpreted as response levels as opposed to thresholds. Appropriate comments will be entered on the bottom of the form. Letters should be written to the referral source and/or school if appropriate.

Billing:
Bill one Pediatric Assessment (Visual Reinforcement Audiometry-CPT 92579 or Conditioned Play Audiometry-CPT 92587) for each 15-minute unit of time involving two clinicians. For one clinician, bill appropriate number of units of Audiogram (CPT 92552 or 92553), Tympanometry (CPT 92567), Acoustic Reflex (CPT 92568), and Consultation (CPT 99242). Bill Clinic Visit (CPT 99211, 99212, or 99213).

References:

Coplan, J. (1993). *Early Language Milestone Scale.* Austin: Pro-Ed.

Glattke, T. J., & Kujawa, S. G. (1991). Otoacoustic emissions. *American Journal of Audiology, 1,* 29-40.

Glattke, T. J., Pafitis, I. A., Cummiskey, C., & Herer, G. R. (1995). Identification of hearing loss in children and young adults using measures of transient otoacoustic emission reproducibility. *American Journal of Audiology, 4,* 67-82.

Hodgson, W. R. (1987). Tests of hearing -- The infant. In F. N. Martin (Ed.), *Hearing Disorders in Children* (pp. 185-216). Austin, TX: Pro-Ed.

Roeser, R. J., & Yellin, W. (1987). Pure-tone tests with preschool children. In F. N. Martin (Ed.), *Hearing Disorders in Children* (pp. 217-264). Austin: Pro-Ed.

Northern, J. L., & Downs, M. P. (1991). *Hearing in Children.* Baltimore: Williams & Wilkins.

Wilson, W. R., & Richardson, M. A. (1991). Behavioral audiometry. In J. D. Osguthorpe and U. Melnick (Eds.), *The Otolaryngologic Clinics of North America* (pp. 285-297). Philadelphia: W. B. Saunders Company.

Protocol 4 Appendix

A.   Pediatric History
B.   Pediatric Historical Review
C.   Services for Hearing Impaired Children

PEDIATRIC HISTORY

DATE

CHILD'S NAME	AGE	GRADE

PARENT'S NAME(S)

WHO REFERRED YOU TO US?

DESCRIBE YOUR CHILD'S PROBLEM:

DO YOU HAVE CONCERNS ABOUT HOW YOUR CHILD HEARS?
DESCRIBE:
    DOES YOUR CHILD:
      a. Respond if you call him/her from another room?   ❑ Yes ❑ No
      b. Respond to his/her name?   ❑ Yes ❑ No
      c. Try to look toward the sound source when a noise is made?   ❑ Yes ❑ No
      d. Alert to familiar sounds - for example a spoon in a cup?   ❑ Yes ❑ No
      e. Stop what he/she is doing when there is an unfamiliar sound? ❑ Yes ❑ No

DO YOU HAVE ANY CONCERNS ABOUT HOW YOUR CHILD TALKS?
DESCRIBE:
    DOES YOUR CHILD:
      a. Say at least 10 words?   ❑ Yes ❑ No
      b. Say 2-3 word sentences?   ❑ Yes ❑ No
      c. Speak clearly to the family?   ❑ Yes ❑ No

NAME OF CHILD'S SCHOOL:

DO YOU HAVE CONCERNS ABOUT YOUR CHILD'S BEHAVIOR (TANTRUMS, HITTING, WILL NOT
FOLLOW DIRECTIONS, ETC.) AT SCHOOL, HOME OR IN THE NEIGHBORHOOD?
DESCRIBE:

IS YOUR CHILD HAVING ANY PROBLEMS LEARNING AT SCHOOL?
DESCRIBE:

DO YOU NOTE ANY PROBLEMS WITH YOUR CHILD'S GENERAL DEVELOPMENT?
DESCRIBE:

AT APPROXIMATELY WHAT AGE DID YOUR CHILD:
    a. Roll over   c. Crawl   e. Say his/her first word
    b. Sit up   d. Walk   f. Toilet train

ARE THERE ANY PROBLEMS WITH YOUR CHILD'S GENERAL HEALTH (PLEASE INCLUDE EAR
INFECTION HISTORY)?
DESCRIBE:

PEDIATRIC HISTORICAL REVIEW

DATE

CHILD'S NAME

FATHER'S NAME   AGE   OCCUPATION
MOTHER'S NAME   AGE   OCCUPATION

WHO HAS ALREADY EVALUATED YOUR CHILD
      Date   Name   Results

HEARING AND AUDITORY INFORMATION
1. Is hearing loss suspected?   At what age? Does the loss fluctuate?

2. Does the child respond to loud noise (airplanes)?   Doorbell or phone?
        Speech over the phone?   Speech when facing the speaker?
        Speech with back to the speaker?   Speech from another room?
        Whispered speech?   Faint sounds?

3. Does the child locate the direction of sound?   4. Does the child watch the speakers face?

5. Does the child wear a hearing aid?   Type?   Age initiated?

SPEECH AND LANGUAGE INFORMATION
1. Did you child babble and then stop?   2. Does your child have a normal voice quality?

3. Give an example of a typical sentence.

4. What is your child's mean length of utterance?   Amount of vocabulary?
     Intelligibility to yourself or others?

5. How are wants expressed?

6. Has there been any change in your child's speech and language development?

7. How much does your child understand?   Nothing?   Gestures?
        With context present?   One stage commands?   etc.?

GENERAL BEHAVIOR INFORMATION
1. Does you child play well with other children?   Cry often?   Have temper tantrums?

2. What are your child's favorite activities or toys?

3. Any special fears?

4. Is behavior consistent from day to day?   Situation to situation?

PEDIATRIC HISTORICAL REVIEW *page 2*

5. Does you child "hear what he wants to hear"?

6. Describe you child's personality (outgoing, cooperative, withdrawn, etc.)?

7. What factors are related to your child's problem (hearing, speech, emotions, brain injury, sibling rivalry, personality, behavioral problems, neglect by either parent, too much protectiveness, mental retardation, inconsistency of parental handling, etc.)?

SCHOOL INFORMATION
1. School attended?   Special services?
         Address:
2. Subjects in which the child excels?   Has difficulty?

3. Grades repeated?

4. Teacher-child relationships?

5. Classroom teacher?   Grade?

DEVELOPMENTAL INFORMATION
1. Did the baby have difficulty sucking, swallowing, or feeding?

2. Describe balance and coordination.

3. Has there been an change in your child's progression of development?

HEALTH INFORMATION
1. Describe general health.

2. Describe significant illnesses (measles, mumps, pneumonia, frequent ear infection, frequent colds, etc.)

3. High fevers?   4. Seizures?

5. Accidents, falls, unconscious, hit in the head or ear?

6. Vision problems?   7. Allergies

8. What medication/s is your child taking?

9. Does your child eat well?   Sleep well?   Have nightmares?   Wet the bed?

PEDIATRIC HISTORICAL REVIEW *page 3*

PREGNANCY AND DELIVERY
1. Condition of the mother's health during pregnancy?   Illnesses, accidents or blood incompatibility (e.g.s.,Toxoplasmosis, Syphilis, Rubella, Cytomegalovirus, and Herpes Simplex Virus)?

2. Length of pregnancy?   Length of labor?   3.   Birth weight (< 1,500 grams-3.3 lbs.)?

4. Type of delivery (normal, induced, breech, caesarean, use of forceps, etc.)

5. Were injuries, scars or deformities noted (defects of the head and neck)?

6. Were there any complications (difficulty breathing (anoxia), jaundiced (requiring exchange transfusion), etc.)

FAMILY INFORMATION
1. Describe hearing problems in other relatives?

2. Are there speech or learning problems in the family?

3. Has there been mental illness, epilepsy or alcoholism in the family?

4. What language is spoken in the home?

5. Are there any problems with other siblings?

SERVICES FOR HEARING IMPAIRED CHILDREN

Issues:
1.   Financial concerns in obtaining amplification

2.   Informational needs on hearing and hearing impairment

3.   Personal concerns in adjusting to a child with a hearing impairment, and the child's adjustment to his or her hearing impairment

4.   Educational concerns relative to placement and remediation considerations

<u>Financial Services</u>
Present the available services to every family. Never assume that a family can afford a hearing aid by the clothes they wear.
1.   Medical Assistance (similar to adults)

2.   Tefra (similar to medical assistance, but it is used for a child with a lot of medical problems. The child is covered, but not the family)

3.   Minnesota Children with Special Health Needs (MCSHN)
        *This organization is state-run and provides free assessments, when prearranged, for any child regardless of the family's income. They will pay for any medical assessment not covered by insurance, with the only exception being psychological assessments. Sometimes if called the day of the assessment, they will still cover the costs.
        *They will cover the cost of hearing aids completely, with a cost-share, or not at all, depending on the family's income.
        *If the family qualifies, MCSHN uses the medical assistance hearing aid contract list.
        *Call MCSHN and give them the child's demographic information. Also, send them a report. The counselor serving the child's county will then contact the family.

4.   Crippled Child Relief
        This organization is privately run with funds acquired by women volunteering their time selling at department stores. The MCSHN counselor will usually direct the family to Crippled Child Relief if they do not qualify for MCSHN services. They usually take the smallest of three bids.

5.   Local services clubs.
        It is most effective if family members contact local service clubs directly, particularly if they know someone in the club.

6.   If the child is older, direct them to the Vocational Rehabilitation part of the Division of Rehabilitation Services. They use the Medical Assistance contract list.

<u>Informational Services</u>
Minnesota Foundation for Better Hearing and Speech (MFBHS) has a very extensive parent package of information, and it is free to the family. With the parents permission, contact MFBHS to have the package sent to the family.

SERVICES FOR HEARING IMPAIRED CHILDREN *page 2*

<u>Educational Services</u>

1.   Send a copy of the results and recommendations to the special education coordinator in the patient's school district. This should be for any age child, as the new federal law mandates service for age of identification.

2.   Contact the educational audiologist by phone to inform them of the child and ask for their assistance in facilitating program placement.

3.   If the parents of severely hearing impaired children are interested in doing some rehabilitation at home, direct them to the John Tracy Clinic correspondence course.

4.   If the child is nearing completion of high school, direct them to the Vocational Rehabilitation portion of the Division of Rehabilitation Services.

Protocol 5
Pediatric Central Auditory Processing Evaluation

Target Population:
Children age 4 to 18 years with normal hearing (PTA ≤ 20 dB HL), but reported difficulty understanding speech in the classroom and in other situations, and those at-risk for academic problems due to suspected auditory processing problems.

Contraindications for formal tests:

1. English is not the primary language.

2. Performance (non-verbal) IQ scores of < 85.

3. Testing is also contraindicated in children with severe speech-language delay, articulation disorder, or psychiatric disorder if the patient is unable to comply with directions, or responses cannot be understood.

4. Significant hearing loss complicates assessment and is often a sufficient explanation for the reported hearing difficulty. However, in situations for which the reported hearing difficulty is out of proportion to the degree of hearing loss, assessment may be carried out if there is no more than mild hearing loss (eg. < 30 dB HL 3-frequency average).

5. In cases of asymmetric loss (interaural 3-frequency average difference ≥ 15 dB HL), binaural and dichotic tests should not be used. Monaural sensitized speech tests may be useful in these cases.

Rationale:
Identification and categorization of central auditory processing problems can allow proper referral to appropriate special education resources, initiation of aural rehabilitation therapy, and provision of assistive listening devices. Counseling parents and teachers regarding results can prevent criticism of the child for poor listening behavior by promoting understanding of the cause of listening problems. When neurologic problems are suspected, referral can be made to pediatric neurology/neuropsychology.

Equipment Required:
Clinical audiometer (pure tone and speech capabilities)
Cassette tape player
Compact disc player
Parent and teacher questionnaires
Recorded speech materials and manuals for central auditory assessment:
- SCAN or SCAN-A Tests for Auditory Processing Disorders (Keith, 1986, 1994a)
- Auditory Continuous Performance Test (Keith, 1994b)
- Pediatric Speech Intelligibility Test (Jerger & Jerger, 1984)
- Tonal and Speech Materials for Auditory Perceptual Assessment (VA-CD)
(Wilson, 1992)

Methods:

At the time an appointment is made for CAP evaluation, a Parent Questionnaire (Appendix A) will be mailed, soliciting history information and requesting details concerning auditory difficulties. A cover letter to the parent(s) will request copies of the child's Individualized Education Plan (IEP), if applicable, and any previous audiologic, educational, psychological, neurologic, and medical evaluations. Additionally, parents will be asked to have the child's teachers complete the Teacher's Questionnaire (Appendix B), and the SIFTER. Other teacher questionnaires may include Fisher's Auditory Problems Checklist (Educational Audiology Association) or the CHAPPS (Smoski, et al., 1992).

The CAP evaluation includes:
   a. Case History
   b. Basic Hearing Evaluation (Protocol 1 or 4)
   c. Speech and Non-Speech Central Auditory Tests
   d. Consultation with child, parents and educational staff

1.   <u>Case History</u>. Through interview with the parent(s), obtain a detailed history of the nature of the auditory problems and any associated educational or social problems. Use the parent questionnaire (Appendix A) as a starting point, and clarify or elaborate upon it as necessary. Use judgement as to whether to include the child in the interview. If the parent is not critical of the child in his or her presence, the process will be less mysterious to the child if he or she is present throughout. Older children will benefit by contributing their own perspective on the problem.

2.   <u>Basic Hearing Evaluation</u>. (Protocol 1 or 4). Unless completed within the last 3 months air, bone, speech and immittance testing including acoustic reflex thresholds will be performed. If the patient has a history of conductive or other fluctuating hearing loss, air, and if necessary, bone conduction thresholds should be repeated. Word recognition testing will be completed in quiet at 30-40 dB re: PTA using a word list appropriate for age (see Pediatric Hearing Evaluation, Protocol 4).

3.   <u>Speech and Non-Speech Central Auditory Tests</u>. Calibrate both channels of the speech audiometer to the tape, and administer according to standardized instructions (refer to pertinent test manual).
   a. Administer a Basic Battery, consisting of:
   - SCAN: A Screening Test for Auditory Processing Disorders, for ages 5-11 years
   - SCAN-A: A Test For Auditory Processing Disorders in Adolescents and Adults, for age 12 years and above
   - Masking Level Difference (MLD) for spondees from the VA Auditory Perceptual Materials CD
   - Auditory Continuous Performance Test (ACPT) to screen for Attention Deficit Disorder.
   - Pitch Pattern Sequence Test (VA CD)
   If all tests are within normal limits, conclude assessment and provide counseling (Step 4.) If tests are abnormal, add supplementary tests from list below, targeted to areas indicated during interview or on questionnaire. For example, if complaints centered on background noise or reverberant environments, choose the time compressed speech with reverberation subtest from the VA Compact Disc. If complaints centered on reading/phonics problems, use the dichotic CV test or the dichotic digits test.
   b. Supplementary Tests:

    - Time Compressed Speech in Reverberation (VA CD)
    - Dichotic CV Test (VA CD)
    - Dichotic Digits Test (VA CD)
Note: the VA compact disc materials are not generally norm-referenced in children. Interpret cautiously, and avoid use in children under 8 years of age.
If the child has articulation errors that make the verbal response mode difficult to interpret, or child's attention is too poor for the verbal response mode (e.g. for 4-5 year-olds), substitute closed-set picture-pointing tests for the Basic Battery.
c. Alternative Closed-Set Test Battery - picture pointing response mode.
- Pediatric Speech Intelligibility Test (Ipsilateral and Contralateral Competing Words and Sentences), normed for ages 3-6
- Selective Auditory Attention Test, normed for ages 4-8

If speech in noise tests were abnormal and consistent with parent/teacher-reported observations, an FM system demonstration may be useful to the parents and child.
d. FM system demonstration for speech recognition in noise. Use minimal amplification settings (SPL ≤ 115 dB, volume set at comfortable level). Test word recognition using W-22, NU-6, PBK or NU-CHIPS lists at signal to noise ratios (S/N) of 0 and -10 dB, with words presented through a sound-field speaker at 0 degrees azimuth, and noise at 90 degrees azimuth (to the ear that will be aided). With the FM system set at a comfortable listening volume and the teacher microphone suspended in front of the 0 degree speaker, repeat measurements with a second word list.

4.   <u>Counseling</u>. If preliminary results are clear, provide initial counseling to review the tests performed and discuss indications for further assessment, referral to another specialty area, or recommendations for intervention/follow-up. Provide additional information, such as classroom suggestions (Appendix C) and General Information Sheet (Appendix D), as appropriate.

Report Format:
Audiologic test results will be entered on the Audiologic Record Form (see Protocol 1). Results of CAP tests will be recorded on their appropriate score forms, and the originals will be kept in a separate CAP file. A report will be written including results of all tests (See sample report, Appendix E). The original CAP report will be placed in the medical chart, and copies will be sent to the referral source, to the parents and to other appropriate parties (e.g., school, pediatrician, other professionals involved in the child's care) as requested by the parents.

Billing:
Bill Audiologic Evaluation as described in Protocol 1 or 4. Bill Central Auditory Processing testing (CPT 92589); 1 unit per 10 minutes of actual testing time under Central Auditory Function. Bill consultation time if counseling is 15 minutes or longer (CPT 99242), 1 unit per 15 minutes.

References:
Cherry, R. S. (1980). *Selective Auditory Attention Test*. Auditec of St. Louis, St. Louis, Missouri.

Fisher, L. *Fisher's Auditory Problems Checklist*. Distributed by the Educational Audiology Association, c/o Utah State University Dept. Communicative Disorders, Logan, Utah, 84322.

Jerger, S., & Jerger, J. (1984). *Pediatric Speech Intelligibility Test.* Auditec of St. Louis, Missouri.

Keith, R. W., Rudy, J., Donahue, P. A., & Katbamna, B. (1989). Comparison of SCAN results with other auditory and language measures in a clinical population. *Ear and Hearing, 10,* 382-386.

Keith, R. W. (1986). *SCAN: A Screening Test for Auditory Processing Disorders.* San Antonio, TX: Psychological Corporation, Harcourt Brace Javonovich, Inc.

Keith, R. W. (1994a). *SCAN-A: A Test For Auditory Processing Disorders in Adolescents and Adults.* San Antonio, TX: Psychological Corporation, Harcourt Brace Javonovich, Inc.

Keith, R. W. (1994b). *ACPT: Auditory Continuous Performance Test.* San Antonio, TX: Psychological Corporation, Harcourt Brace Javonovich, Inc.

Mueller, H. G., & Bright, K. E. (1994). Monosyllabic procedures in central testing. In J. Katz (Ed.), *Handbook of Clinical Audiology* (pp. 222-238). Baltimore, MD: Williams & Wilkins.

Noffsinger, D., Martinez, C. D., & Wilson, R. H. (1994a). Dichotic listening to speech: Background and preliminary data for digits, sentences, and nonsense syllables. *Journal of the American Academy of Audiology, 5,* 248-254.

Noffsinger, D., Wilson, R. H., & Musiek, F. E. (1994b). Department of Veterans Affairs compact disc recording for auditory perceptual assessment: Background and introduction. *Journal of the American Academy of Audiology, 5,* 231-235.

Schoeny, Z. G., & Talbott, R. E. (1994). Nonspeech procedures in central testing. In J. Katz (Ed.), *Handbook of Clinical Audiology* (pp. 212-221). Baltimore, MD: Williams & Wilkins.

Smoski, W. J., Brunt, M.A., and Tannahill, J.C. (1992). Listening characteristics of children with central auditory processing disorders. *Language, Speech and Hearing Services in the Schools,* 23, 145-152.

Willeford, J., & Burleigh, J. (1985). *Handbook of Central Auditory Processing Disorders in Children.* New York: Grune and Stratton.

Wilson, R. H. (1992). *Tonal and Speech Materials for Auditory Perceptual Assessment.* Department of Veteran's Affairs, Produced by Auditory Research Laboratories, VA Medical Centers Long Beach and West Los Angeles, California and Dartmouth-Hitchcock Medical Center, Wharon, New Hampshire.

Wilson, R. H., Preece, J. P., Salamon, D. L., Sperry, J. L., & Bornstein, S. P. (1994a). Effects of time compression and time compression plus reverberation on the intelligibility of NU auditory test no. 6. *Journal of the American Academy of Audiology, 5 ,* 269-277.

Wilson, R. H., Zizz, C. A., & Sperry, J. L. (1994b). Masking level difference for spondaic words in 2000-msec bursts of broadband noise. *Journal of the American Academy of Audiology, 5,* 236-242.

Protocol 5 Appendix

A.   Parent's Questionnaire: Children's Hearing Speech/Language History
B.   Teacher's Questionnaire: Auditory, Academic & Social Profile
C.   Improving Listening Environment in the Classroom
D.   General Information for Parents and Teachers About Auditory Processing Disorders
E.   A Sample Report of an Auditory Processing Evaluation

PARENT'S QUESTIONNAIRE
CHILDREN'S HEARING, SPEECH/LANGUAGE HISTORY

The information you provide in this questionnaire will help us assess your child's auditory processing capabilities properly. Please fill out this form, answering questions about your child, as completely as possible. If there are any items you do not fully understand, discuss them with your child's audiologist during the appointment.

IDENTIFYING INFORMATION

Child's Name		Birthdate	Sex	Age
Person Completing Form:		Date	Daytime Phone	
Address			Evening Phone	
City	State		Zip	

REASON(S) FOR TESTING (check all which apply)

	Academic		Speech / Language Problems		Attention Problems
	Hearing		Reading / Phonics Problems		Other:

HOME AND FAMILY INFORMATION

Father's Name	Occupation
Last grade completed in school	Age
Mother's Name	Occupation
Last grade completed in school	Age
Child lives with:	Languages spoken in home:

OTHER CHILDREN IN THE FAMILY

Name	Age	Sex	Grade Level	List any speech, hearing, learning or medical problems

BIRTH HISTORY	Yes	No	BIRTH HISTORY	Yes	No
Prenatal Problems			Ventilation used		
Prenatal Alcohol Exposure			Neonatal infection		
Prenatal Drug Exposure			Meningitis		
Premature Birth			Herpes		
Blood incompatibility			Cytomegalovirus		
Blood transfusion			Toxoplasmosis		
Baby in intensive care			Rubella		
Apgar Scores:			Birthweight:		

PARENT'S QUESTIONNAIRE *page 2*

MEDICAL HISTORY	Yes	No	Date Occurred	Description
Current Medical Conditions				
Taking Medications				
Head injuries				
Convulsions				
Headaches				
Serious infections				
Other brain/spinal problems				
Surgeries				

HEARING AND EAR HISTORY	Description
Do you think your child's hearing is poor?	
Does your child complain of noises in the ears or head?	
Does your child have dizziness or imbalance?	
Age at first ear infection (nurse or doctor diagnosed)	
Number of ear infections age 0-2 years	
Number of ear infections age 2-4 years	
Number of ear infections age 4-6 years	
Last ear infection (date or age)	
Ear surgeries (ages, ear operated on and type of surgery)	
Has child used hearing aids?	

TESTS DONE	Where	Date	Age	Results
Hearing Test				
Speech/Language				
Vision Exam				
Neurological (EEG)				
Psychological				
CT Scan or MRI				

FAMILY HISTORY	Description (relationship to child and type of problem)
Neurologic diseases	
Speech problems	
Learning problems	
Hereditary illness	
Ear/hearing	

PARENT'S QUESTIONNAIRE *page 3*

SOCIAL / EMOTIONAL	YES	NO		YES	NO
Trouble understanding television programs			Appears confused in noisy places		
Sensitivity to loud sounds			Often says "huh" or "what"		
Trouble telling where sounds are			Mixes up sounds		
Problems following directions			Needs quiet to study		
Easily distracted			Restless		
Daydreams			Problem sitting still		
Forgetful			Rowdiness		
Preference for playing with younger children			Preference for playing with older children		
Disruptive			Headaches		
Preference for solitary activities			Short attention span		
Lacks motivation			Temper tantrums		
Easily frustrated			Easily flustered or confused		
Tires easily			Hyperactive		
Often tense or anxious			Disobedient		
Uncooperative			Shy		
Clumsy			Irritable		
Impulsive			Destructive		
Lacks self-confidence			Excessive talking		
Easily upset by new situations			Seeks attention		
Has problems with time concept			Does not complete assignments		
Fakes illnesses			Dislikes school		
Underachiever			Problems with the law		
Involved with drugs			Involved with alcohol		
Please explain further items checked above:					

PARENT'S QUESTIONNAIRE *page 4*

SPEECH / LANGUAGE PROBLEMS	Yes	No	Description
Delay in early speech development			
Small vocabulary compared to peers			
Poor grammar usage			
Problem speaking clearly			
Stuttering			
Problem understanding others			
Speech therapy now or in past			

SCHOOL / EDUCATIONAL INFORMATION	
School currently attending	Grade in school
Best subject(s)	Has child received chapter 1 help?
Receives speech therapy	Receives other therapy
Poorest subject(s)	Has your child ever repeated a grade?
Does child have an IEP?	Does your child like school?

Are you satisfied with school support? If no, please explain:

Has your child's teacher ever expressed concern for your child's progress? If yes, please explain:

WHO SHOULD RECEIVE A COPY OF THE EVALUATION REPORT ?		
Name	Address	Phone

Thank you for your time and effort filling out this questionnaire.

TEACHER'S QUESTIONNAIRE
AUDITORY, ACADEMIC & SOCIAL PROFILE

Child _____ Grade _____ School _____

Observer _____ Position _____ Date _____

On a scale of 1 (never) to 5 (always), rate the student's difficulty with the following:

		Never	Occasionally	Often	Usually	Always
1.	Has difficulty in paying attention to speaker	1	2	3	4	5
2.	Is a poor listener	1	2	3	4	5
3.	Disturbed by background noise	1	2	3	4	5
	SPECIFICALLY:					
	a. speech	1	2	3	4	5
	b. whispering	1	2	3	4	5
	c. shuffling papers, feet, etc.	1	2	3	4	5
	d. pencil sharpener	1	2	3	4	5
	e. playground noise	1	2	3	4	5
	f. from other classrooms or halls	1	2	3	4	5
	g. other (class bells, etc.)	1	2	3	4	5
4.	Daydreams	1	2	3	4	5
5.	Has short attention span	1	2	3	4	5
6.	Misunderstands verbal instructions	1	2	3	4	5
7.	Misunderstands written instructions	1	2	3	4	5
8.	Asks for repetition of verbal instructions	1	2	3	4	5
9.	Slow or delayed response to verbal stimuli	1	2	3	4	5
10.	Has trouble recalling verbal material	1	2	3	4	5

TEACHER'S QUESTIONNAIRE   *page 2*

ACADEMIC PROFILE	Never	Occasionally	Often	Usually	Always
1. Decreased performance in:	1	2	3	4	5
Mathematics	1	2	3	4	5
Reading	1	2	3	4	5
Spelling	1	2	3	4	5
Phonics	1	2	3	4	5
Language Arts	1	2	3	4	5
Other _____	1	2	3	4	5
2. Slow starter	1	2	3	4	5
3. Difficulty completing tasks	1	2	3	4	5
4. Relies heavily on visual cues in classroom	1	2	3	4	5
5. Receives resource-tutorial help	1	2	3	4	5
6. Receives speech/language therapy	1	2	3	4	5

SOCIAL PROFILE	Never	Occasionally	Often	Usually	Always
1. Impulsive	1	2	3	4	5
2. Frustrated	1	2	3	4	5
3. Withdrawn	1	2	3	4	5
4. Aggressive	1	2	3	4	5
5. Not accepted by peers	1	2	3	4	5
6. Prefers association with younger children	1	2	3	4	5
7. Child is a "loner"	1	2	3	4	5
8. Restless/excessive physical movement	1	2	3	4	5
9. Disturbs other children during class	1	2	3	4	5
10. Gives up easily	1	2	3	4	5
11. Seeks assistance from teacher	1	2	3	4	5
12. Insensitive to time responsibilities	1	2	3	4	5

From: Willeford, J. A., & Burleigh, J. M. (1985). *Handbook of Central Auditory Processing Disorders in Children,* pp. 57- 58.

IMPROVING THE LISTENING ENVIRONMENT IN THE CLASSROOM

• It is critical that each child in the class can hear well in order to learn. The teacher's physical position and the noise both within and outside of the classroom affects how all students hear, and in turn, learn.

• It is estimated that 49% of material in primary grades is presented auditorally, while in middle school, 65% of information is given auditorally. Unfortunately, many classrooms are not well-designed for these listening demands.

• 30% of all students in classrooms studied have short term and/or long-term hearing loss.

• Typical ear infections cause a "plugged ear" hearing loss, and muffled speech. To simulate, plug your ears tightly with your fingertips. Note the distinct difference in speech sounds.

• Children with long-term hearing loss in only one ear have 10 times the risk for failing a grade in school.

• Simple classroom modifications can help ALL students hear better, not just those with hearing problems. Effective classroom teaching styles that help children with hearing loss also benefit other children.

• Classroom amplification systems have been shown to benefit all students, but especially those with minimal hearing loss, learning disabilities, attention deficit disorders and central auditory disorders. Teachers consistently rate these systems highly for classroom control and less vocal fatigue. These systems are also highly cost-effective, considering that they assist more than one student and last for years.

SOURCES OF NOISE IN CLASSROOMS

Room Occupant Noise

-Coughing, sneezing

-Talking, whispering

-Paper, books, supplies shuffling

-Chair, desk movement

Equipment Noise

-Projectors

-VCRs

-Computers

Doors

-hallway noise

-squeaky hinges

Ventilation

-Fans

-Air conditioners

-Heating ducts

Florescent Light Ballasts

Adjacent Classrooms

Windows

-Playground

-Traffic

-Lawn maintenance

IMPROVING THE LISTENING ENVIRONMENT IN THE CLASSROOM *page 2*

CLASSROOM ACOUSTICS

The two enemies of good acoustics for listening are noise and excess reverberation (echoes). A moderate amount of reverberation gives speech a pleasant boost, but too much causes distortion and difficult listening.   Hard, reflective surfaces increase reverberation.   Sources of reverberation include:

-Hard surface floors
-Reflective, non-porous walls
-Large areas of exposed glass windows
-Chalkboards
-Plaster ceilings
-High ceilings
-Large open areas
-Large furnishings (file cabinets, mirrors, reflective room dividers)

HELPFUL TIPS TO IMPROVE CLASSROOM ACOUSTICS

Floors: Carpet or carpet tiles are excellent sound absorbers. Area rugs (industrial grade is easiest to maintain) are inexpensive and easy to add. Rugs absorb sound as well as reduce foot and chair noise.

Walls: Partial covering of large reflective walls with acoustic tile, cork board, absorbent wall coverings reduce reverberation. Treatment of one of two parallel walls is sufficient.

Windows: Cover large glass windows with fabric curtains. Move students away from windows if possible. Close windows at least partially to reduce outside sound.

Chalkboards: Many classrooms, especially older ones, have far too much board space. Replacement with cork board or wall hangings is helpful.

Ceilings: Absorbent ceiling tiles, especially acoustic tiles, are very helpful. Tiles need many holes or absorbent surfaces to be effective. Ceiling hung fabric panels can also be helpful, but take care that they are not visually distracting.

IMPROVING THE LISTENING ENVIRONMENT IN THE CLASSROOM *page 3*

Sound barriers: Large items such as bookcases, cabinets and room dividers can help shield noisier areas from areas that need quiet. They also help break up large rooms for better acoustics.

Ventilation systems: Ventilator grills with tiny holes restrict air movement and create noise. Replace with larger, non-restricting types. Vibrating sheet metal ductwork can be made less noisy by attaching angle iron supports to them for support.

Florescent lights: Light ballasts can sometimes produce loud buzzing noise; replacement of the ballast can solve this problem.

Equipment noise: Add printer shields to reduce noise from computers. Locate computers near sound absorbing treatments. Select new equipment for its low sound properties.

Doors: Close doors and windows when noise is present outside; suggest rearrangement of noisy activities away from classrooms.

Don't hesitate to ask an educational audiologist for suggestions about your classroom. Small, inexpensive steps can be surprisingly effective.

GENERAL INFORMATION FOR PARENTS AND TEACHERS ABOUT: CENTRAL AUDITORY PROCESSING DISORDERS (CAPD)

What is a central auditory processing disorder?

A Central Auditory Processing problem is the inability or decreased ability to attend to, discriminate, recognize, or understand information that is presented auditorally (by listening). Most language is learned by listening. In order to learn in school, a child must have normal hearing, be able to listen attentively during the school day, and be able to separate out important speech (like yours or the teacher's directions) from all the other noises present at home and at school. When a child's auditory skills are not good, it will be more challenging, and sometimes too difficult to learn without special assistance. Most people with central auditory processing problems have normal intelligence and normal hearing sensitivity.

What are the characteristics of CAPD?

Children with auditory processing problems may have some or all of the following characteristics:
- Respond inconsistently to sound (sometimes they hear and sometimes not)
- Short attention span, especially when asked to listen
- Easily distracted by sounds and visual disturbances
- Have difficulty telling where a sound is coming from
- Become upset by background or loud sounds
- Frequently request that information be repeated
- Have trouble remembering things they have learned auditorally
- Have trouble with phonics
- Have a long or repeated history of otitis media

What causes central auditory processing disorders?

CAPD has several possible causes, although more research is needed to understand the causes. Some are caused by neurological (brain) disorders, birth trauma, meningitis or other viral infections, head trauma, or by a history of hearing loss early in life due to chronic or repeated otitis media (ear infections). Because the brain is maturing rapidly in the first few years of life, auditory input needs to be consistent for the brain to develop pathways normally. Uncorrected hearing loss may cause delay in both language and in processing skills in some children, and hearing loss due to repeated ear infections can also contribute to later processing problems. Sometimes, no cause can be determined.

How is a central auditory processing disorder detected?

Usually, a parent or teacher suspects hearing loss because the child is inattentive or inconsistent in responding to sound. The first step when these concerns are expressed is to have a complete basic hearing evaluation by a certified or licensed audiologist. If the hearing evaluation shows normal hearing, it should be followed by special tests that probe the child's ability to hear in difficult conditions, like those experienced at home or school.

GENERAL INFORMATION FOR PARENTS AND TEACHERS ABOUT:
CENTRAL AUDITORY PROCESSING DISORDERS (CAPD) *page 2*

What can be done if my child has auditory processing problems?

Determining just what situations cause trouble, and to what extent the child has trouble is the first step. Following this or at the same time, consultations with speech-language pathologists (who evaluate and treat speech and language problems), neurologists (who evaluate diseases of the nervous system), occupational therapists (who evaluate visual perceptual problems), psychologists (who evaluate intelligence and learning disabilities) may be consulted.

Understand that your child's listening problems are not willful, nor are they the result of behavior problems. Listening skills can improve with careful attention and control of the learning environment. Some children benefit from speech-language therapy, if a delay is detected. Other children may benefit from special listening systems that they wear personally, or that are placed in the classroom. The program for your child must be tailored to his or her specific needs.

REPORT OF AUDITORY PROCESSING EVALUATION

Name: K.O.
UMHC #: 1824825-4
Birthdate: 2/25/88
Address:

Referred By: Dr. M
Reason for Referral: Auditory
Processing Evaluation
Date of Assessment: 2 August 95

BACKGROUND INFORMATION

K is a 7 year-old boy who was referred to evaluate whether his difficulties in phonics, reading, and auditory understanding are related to difficulty processing auditory information. K was accompanied by his mother, Valerie, who provided history through interview and on a written questionnaire. Her primary concerns relate to K's difficulty reading and at times, and hearing what is said to him. K received speech therapy two times a week, and daily Title I resource support last year in Kindergarten. He is progressing this year to first grade. K was seen for Occupational Therapy between December of 1994 and June of 1995 to improve fine motor skills and daily living skills. He was discharged from therapy in July as he made adequate progress in these areas.

K's mother reports normal pregnancy and delivery, with no birth complications. K was small for gestational age, at 4 lbs., 11 oz., but all 4 of her children were in this range at birth. K has 3 older sisters. Developmental milestones (walking, sitting, babbling, following directions) were reached at normal ages. No medical problems reported, and no family history of neurologic, learning or hearing problems were noted. K has normal intellectual function (Full-scale IQ = 101), but his verbal IQ score was 15 points below his performance IQ score. K's mother has questioned his hearing ability. He is sensitive to loud sounds, and has a history of recurrent otitis media beginning at 6-9 months, and continuing episodically through age 4. Mom reports that K has trouble localizing sounds and following directions at times, is easily distracted and daydreams, seems confused in noisy places to the point of becoming tense, and needs quiet to read. A teacher questionnaire filled out by _____, Primary School, indicates the following areas of concern: Math, reading, phonics, relies heavily on visual cues in classroom.

EVALUATION RESULTS

Test Behavior :

K easily separated from his mother for testing, and cooperated with all tests. He was very quiet and attentive during testing, but tended to mumble responses at times. He responded well to verbal praise for attention to the task. These results are felt to be reliable indicators of K's auditory abilities.

Tests of Hearing Sensitivity and Middle Ear Function :

Hearing sensitivity for pure tones was normal in both ears. Word understanding (repetition of words in quiet) showed normal speech perception ability under ideal conditions (score 100% for both ears).

REPORT OF AUDITORY PROCESSING EVALUATION *page 2*

Tympanometry showed normal peak pressure and admittance for both ears, reflecting normal middle ear function. Acoustic reflex thresholds were normal in both ears, indicating grossly normal auditory brainstem function.

SCAN Battery :
This test screens ability to perceive speech that is degraded due to background noise, filtering, or due to competition from other speech.

Subtest	Raw Score	Standard Score	Percentile Rank
Filtered Words	37	14	91%
Auditory Figure-Ground	35	13	84%
Competing Words	39	4	2%
SCAN Composite	111	81	10%

Competing words: Analysis of ear dominance :
Right-ear-first = 17 to right (prevalence = 2%)
Left-ear-first = 17 to right (prevalence = <1%)

Interpretation: K's overall performance fell below average, at 1 standard deviation below the mean. Filtered words, which assesses auditory closure, showed above average performance. Auditory figure ground, which assesses ability to perceive speech in background speech noise also showed above average performance. Competing words, however, which assess maturation of the auditory pathways, showed very low scores, at the 2nd percentile. Of note was that K showed a strong, consistent right ear dominance, consistent with immaturity of the central auditory nervous system.

Masking Level Difference (MLD):
This test assesses how well both ears work together to suppress competing noise. Two-syllable words were given to both ears at 50 dB HL with broadband noise in phase at both ears. Words were then presented with noise out of phase at the left relative to the right ear, which provides a cue to suppress the noise. The MLD was measured at 4.5 dB (normal range ≥ 5 dB).

Interpretation: The MLD test indicated decreased ability to suppress noise when using both ears together.

Dichotic Digits:
This test measures ability to hear and repeat simultaneous speech. Digits are generally more easily perceived and more predictable than words, as in the competing words portion of the SCAN. Dichotic digits recorded on compact disc were presented at 50 dB HL with simultaneous onset at both ears. Performance was 94% for the right ear and 39% for the left ear. There was a significant right ear advantage, consistent with results from the SCAN. This finding further suggests immaturity of the central auditory nervous system.

REPORT OF AUDITORY PROCESSING EVALUATION *page 3*

SUMMARY AND RECOMMENDATIONS

K's hearing sensitivity was normal for both tones and speech in quiet. That is, K is able to hear well under ideal conditions. However, his auditory processing profile shows significant auditory processing problems under complex listening situations. For example, when he has to listen to two meaningful messages at once, he is unable to do so effectively and a strong advantage for his right ear emerges. In real-life situations, this means that K may have trouble with complex tasks (for example, multi-step directions) or divided attention tasks.

It is not uncommon for children with auditory processing problems to also have speech-language delay and reading difficulties, as K does. These may be related issues, reflecting immaturity of auditory-language skills. K will benefit from a coordinated program to address all three areas (language, reading, and audition).

(1) For the auditory problems, one effective approach is to try to help K adopt compensation strategies, to allow him to learn to use his hearing more effectively for learning, and to use other senses (vision, tactile) to compensate for the weaker auditory system.

(2) Specific strategies that may benefit K are enclosed with this report. However, every child, teacher, and classroom environment is different.

(3) I recommend that a hearing consultant from the Special Education Coop be asked to assess K's listening skills in his learning environment, and depending on specific problems uncovered, the hearing consultant can suggest strategies to K's teacher to adapt the environment or teaching to allow better hearing in the classroom.

(4) Re-evaluation in one to two years (or as necessary for IEP planning) is recommended to assess maturation and continued need for accommodations in the classroom.

If the reader of this report has any questions regarding these test results or the recommendations given, please contact me at XXX-XXXX.

Audiologist

cc: Referring Physician
       Occupational Therapist
       Teacher
       Parents
       School Case Manager

Protocol 6 Extended High Frequency Audiometry

Target Population:
Patients at risk for high frequency hearing loss. This group includes, but is not limited to patients receiving:
- chemotherapy
- renal dialysis
- ototoxic medications (see Appendix A)
- patients with severe-profound hearing loss since birth or early childhood, and speech production better than expected based on degree of loss in conventional frequencies
- patients with tinnitus unexplained by hearing loss in conventional frequencies.

Patients suffering from temporary effects of middle ear disease are poor candidates for extended high frequency (EHF) audiometry for purposes of monitoring ototoxic effects. Determination of patients at risk for ototoxicity will follow the definition of risk criteria in the Criteria and Schedule for Monitoring Ototoxic Effects attached as Appendix B. Patients with severe hearing losses with flat or rising configurations may have good EHF hearing and should be tested.

Rationale:
Ototoxically induced hearing losses are thought to initially manifest themselves as an alteration in the function of the Organ of Corti at the basal end of the cochlea. This disease process is evident as a change in the sensitivity of hearing in the extended high frequencies, which appear to be more sensitive to ototoxic effects than conventional frequencies.

Patients with severe-profound hearing loss in conventional frequencies and relatively good speech production may have usable residual hearing in the extended high frequencies. Because they could potentially benefit from frequency transposition hearing aids, they should be tested in the EHF range.

Hearing thresholds above 8 kHz are strongly age dependent and intersubject variability is higher in this range (see Appendix C). Test-retest variability within a subject is substantially smaller than variation between subjects. For this reason, a pre-treatment baseline is the best method to determine if change occurs in conjunction with chemotherapy or other potentially ototoxic medications. Determination of hearing loss at higher frequencies is based on comparisons of a patient's hearing thresholds at baseline and after treatment with suspected ototoxic agents. Criteria for significant change are listed under Methods.

Equipment Required:
Extended high frequency audiometer
Koss Pro/4x earphones

Methods:

A baseline evaluation consisting of a basic hearing evaluation (Protocol 1) and extended high frequency audiometric testing should be completed on the initial visit. Cerumen removal (Protocol 3) should be performed for patients who are discovered to have 50% or greater cerumen occlusion upon otoscopic examination, or for those patients in which the cerumen prevents otoscopic visualization of the eardrum.

Thresholds should be obtained for frequencies 8, 10, 12.5, 16, and 20 kHz using the method described in ANSI S3.21 (1978) American National Standard Methods for Manual Puretone Threshold Audiometry. Additional frequencies (9, 11.2, 14, and 18 kHz) shall also be tested whenever the thresholds differ by 20 dB or more between the test frequencies below 12.5 kHz, or by 40 dB or more between frequencies above 12.5 kHz. The next lower frequency should be tested in cases where thresholds cannot be obtained at the maximum stimulus level (typically 115 dB SPL). Masking should be applied to the ear opposite the test ear whenever the unmasked interaural threshold difference equals or exceeds 30 dB.

Ideally, baseline audiograms should be obtained before initiating treatment. However, audiograms can be accepted as baseline if they are obtained within 48 hours of the beginning of the treatment course. They should be clearly labeled as baseline data (see Appendix D).

Repeat testing generally follows the schedule set forth in Criteria and Schedule of Monitoring Ototoxic Effects (see Appendix B). Chemotherapy patients should be retested before the administration of each therapy session, or sooner if the patient has hearing concerns, tinnitus or dizziness. Retests include basic and extended high frequency pure tone thresholds. If appropriate, include speech recognition testing and tympanometry.

Criteria for significant threshold shift: Compare current findings to baseline or most recent test.

8 - 12.5 kHz:	10 dB or greater difference at two or more frequencies.
14 - 20 kHz:	20 dB or greater difference at two or more frequencies.

Report Format:

The extended high frequency audiometric evaluations are reported in the patient chart using the High Frequency Audiometry Form (see Appendix E). In the report indicate how the results relate to the patient's age norms (see Appendix C) and to previous test results.

Billing:

Bill Air Conduction (CPT 92552); one unit per ear tested.

References:

American National Standards Institute. (1978). *American National Standard Methods for Manual Pure-Tone Threshold Audiometry.* (ANSI S3.21 - 1978). New York.

Ahonen, J. E., & McDermott, J. C. (1984). Extended high frequency hearing loss in children with cleft palate. *Audiology, 23,* 467-476.

Dreschler, W. A., v.d. Hulst, R. J. A. M., Tange, R. A., & Urbanus, N. A. M. (1985). The role of high-frequency audiometry in early detection of ototoxicity. *Audiology, 24,* 387-395.

Fausti, S. A., Frey, R. H., Henry, J. A., Knutson, J. L., & Olson, D. J. (1990). Reliability and validity of high frequency (8-20 kHz) thresholds obtained on a computer-based audiometer as compared to a documented laboratory system. *Journal of the American Academy of Audiology, 1*, 162 - 170.

Fausti, S. A., Erickson, D. A., Frey, R. H., Rappaport, B. Z., & Schechter, M. A. (1981). The effects of noise upon human hearing sensitivity from 8000 - 20000 Hz. *Journal of the Acoustical Society of America, 69*, 1343 - 1349.

Fausti, S. A., Frey, R. H., Erickson, D. A., Rappaport, B. Z., & Cleary, E. J. (1979). A system for evaluating auditory function from 8000 - 20000 Hz. *Journal of the Acoustical Society of America, 66*, 1713 - 1719.

Hunter, L. L., Margolis, R. H., Rykken, J. R., Le, C. T., Dale, K. A., & Giebink, G. S. (1996). Extended high frequency hearing loss associated with otitis media. *Ear and Hearing, 17*, 1-11.

Margolis, R. H., Hunter, L. L., Saupe, J. R., & Giebink, G. S. (1993). Effects of otitis media on extended high frequency hearing in children. *Annals of Otology Rhinology Laryngology, 102*, 1-5.

Laukli, E., & Mair, I. W. S. (1985). High frequency audiometry: Normative studies and preliminary experiences. *Scandinavian Audiology, 14*, 151-158.

Rappaport, B. Z., Fausti, S. A., Schechter, J. A., & Frey, R. H. (1982). Investigation of interaural attenuation factors for frequencies above 8000 Hz. *Journal of the Acoustical Society of America, 72*, 1297-1298.

Stelmachowicz, P. G., Beauchaine, K. A., Kalberer, A., & Jesteadt, W. (1989). Normative thresholds in the 8 to 20 kHz range as a function of age. *Journal of the Acoustical Society of America, 86*, 1384 - 1391.

Stelmachowicz, P. G., Beauchaine, K. A., Kalberer, A., Kelly, W. J., & Jesteadt, W. (1989). High frequency audiometry: Test reliability & procedural considerations. *Journal of the Acoustical Society of America, 85*, 879 - 887.

Protocol 6 Appendix

A.   Ototoxic Drug List
B.   Criteria and Schedule for Monitoring Ototoxic Effects
C.   Suggested Schedule for Monitoring Renal Function of Patients
      Treated with Aminoglycosides
D.   Mean Thresholds Referenced to the Flat-Plate Coupler
E.   Example of an Extended High Frequency Audiogram

OTOTOXIC DRUG LIST

Aminoglycoside Antibiotics	Other Antibiotics	Other Drugs	Loop Diuretics
amikacin	capreomycin	chloroquine phosphate	bumetinide (bumex)
gentamicin	cephaloridine	cisplatin	ethacrynic acid
kanamycin	cephalothin	fenoprofin	furosemide (lasix)
neomycin	chloramphenicol	ibuprofin	
netilmicin	colistin	naproxen	
paromomycin	erythromycin	nitrogen mustard	
sismicin	minocycline	quinidine	
streptomycin	polymyxin	quinine	
tobramycin	ristocetin	salicylates	
	vancomycin	suldinac	
	viomycin	carboplatin	

AMINOGLYCOSIDE ANTIBIOTICS

GENERAL: (Brand Name)

<u>OTOTOXICITY</u>

-permanent loss of inner and outer hair cells
beginning with basal turn and progressing
to the apex
-ototoxicity related to dosage and combination
with other drugs, renal function, and age
-can have delayed onset
-cochleotoxic and/or vestibulotoxic, including
tinnitus, vertigo, and nausea
-word recognition scores often disproportionately poor
-intrauterine toxicity possible
-if ingested, toxicity unlikely because aminoglycoside
are poorly absorbed from an intact gastro-intestinal tract

<u>USAGE</u>

-treatment of bacterial infections
systemically and topically
-sterilizing agents
-wound irrigation

AMIKACIN: (Amikin)
-cochleotoxic   -staph infections

GENTAMICIN: (Garamycin, G-Myticin)
-vestibulotoxic, dizziness, vertigo, tinnitus   -meningitis
maybe some high frequency hearing loss   -neonatal sepsis
with excessive doses   -bacterial septicemia
                                                     -topical use on burns

KANAMYCIN: (Kantrex)
-cochleotoxic, bilateral high frequency hearing   -tuberculosis
loss may be partially reversible   -peritonitis
-tinnitus, loss of balance

OTOTOXIC DRUG LIST *page 2*

NEOMYCIN:
- -cochleotoxic
- -bilateral high frequency hearing loss reversible or irreversible

- -bacterial infections
- -wound & cavity irrigation
- -renal failure

NETILMICIN:(Netromycin)
- -cochleotoxic

- -bacterial infections

STREPTOMYCIN:
- -vestibulotoxic- nausea, vomiting, vertigo
- -renal impairment predisposes ototoxicity
- -hearing loss only after long term therapy

- -tuberculosis
- -urinary tract infections

TOBRAMYCIN: (Nebcin)
- -bilateral irreversible high frequency hearing loss, vertigo, tinnitus , neurotoxicity

- -bone marrow transplants
- -septicemia, neonatal sepsis

OTHER ANTIBIOTICS

ERYTHROMYCIN: (E-Mycin)
<u>Otoxicity</u>
- -tinnitus, vertigo

<u>Usage</u>
- -treatment of infections

NEOMYCIN: (Neosporin, Cortisporin)
- -ototoxic if used over a wide area (topically) for extended periods of time

- -not to be used in ear canal if ear drum is perforated

VANCOMYCIN: (Vancocin)
- -cochleotoxic
- -may be permanent hearing loss associated with high doses, renal failure, or concurrent use with other ototoxic drugs

- -severe infections
- -septicemia; endocarditis
- -bone infections
- -lower respiratory tract infections
- -skin & structure infections

DIURETICS

GENERAL
- -ototoxic with high doses
- -loss may be sudden and usually reversible
- -usually hearing loss in low/mid range
- -mainly cochleotoxic
- -effects on vestibular system usually temporary

- -edema from kidney failure or coronary failure

BUMETANIDE: (Bumex)
- -potential for ototoxicity exists, however blood levels necessary to produce ototoxicity will be rarely achieved

OTOTOXIC DRUG LIST *page 3*

ETHACRYNIC ACID: (Edecrin)
-reversible hearing loss of short duration   -treatment of edema
-sense of fullness in the ears   -congestive heart failure
-tinnitus and vertigo   -cirrhosis of the liver
-may increase ototoxic potential of other drugs   -renal disorders

FUROSEMIDE: (Lasix)
-reversible or permanent hearing loss   -renal disorders
associated with rapid injection   -dermal infections
-hearing loss also associated with concomitant   -cardiac disorders
therapy with other ototoxic drugs

ANTIMALARIAL

GENERAL:
    Ototoxicity   Usage
-cochleotoxic, tinnitus   -malaria
-hearing loss usually reversible

QUININE: (Quinidex)
-intrauterine ototoxicity   -malaria
-hearing loss associated with high doses

QUINIDINE:
-tinnitus, vertigo, dizziness   -cardiac arrhythmia
-some hearing loss possible

CYTOXICS

GENERAL: Usage
-ototoxicity related to dosage   -chemical treatment of tumors
-hearing loss can be asymmetrical   and malignancies
-hearing loss is permanent
-effects high frequencies first, later affects all frequencies
-can include otalgia and tinnitus
-word recognition scores often disproportionately poor

CIS-PLATINUM: (Platinol)
-tinnitus   -testicular/ovarian cancer
-high frequency hearing loss, uni/bilateral
-ototoxicity if cumulative

NITROGEN MUSTARD: (Mustargen)
-tinnitus and diminished hearing   -lymphocytic leukemia
                                                    -Hodgkin's Disease

CARBO-PLATIN (Paraplatin)
-1% incidence of Hearing loss

OTOTOXIC DRUG LIST *page 4*

ANALGESICS/ANTI-INFLAMMATORY DRUGS

GENERAL:
-ototoxicity with high doses
-usually a flat hearing loss (20 - 40 dB)
-usually preceded by tinnitus
-usually reversible hearing loss

-analgesic, anti-inflammatory use
-rheumatoid/osteo arthritis

CRITERIA AND SCHEDULE FOR MONITORING OTOTOXIC EFFECTS

CRITERIA: Patients who are treated with ototoxic drugs will be classified as **at risk** or **high risk** on the following criteria.

At risk: Patients are at risk for ototoxicity if any of the following conditions are met.
1. Treatment with 1 ototoxic medication (excluding diuretics) for $\geq$ 21 days regardless of peak and trough levels.
2. Treatment with 1 ototoxic medication for $\geq$ 2 days with peak and trough levels exceeding safe ranges on 2 or more occasions.
3. Simultaneous treatment with 2 or more ototoxic medications for $\geq$ 2 days.

High risk: Patients are at high risk for ototoxicity if any of the following conditions are met:
1.   Patient is at risk and had renal impairment (serum creatinine $\geq$ 1.4 mg/100 ml or BUN $\geq$ 30).
2.   Patient is at risk and exhibits symptoms of inner ear disease (tinnitus, hearing loss, dizziness, imbalance, posture disorder).
3.   Patient is at risk and has a family history of hearing impairment.
4.   Simultaneous treatment with 2 or more ototoxic medications for $\geq$ 7 days
5.   Treatment with 1 ototoxic medication with peak and trough levels exceeding safe ranges for 3 successive days.

Schedule and Procedures: Alert patients will be tested by behavioral audiometry. Those who cannot be tested behaviorally will be evaluated by auditory brainstem response (ABR). Sedation will be used if necessary, and not medically contraindicated. A **baseline evaluation** will be obtained as early as possible for at risk patients, consisting of the following tests:

Alert Patients	**Non-Alert Patients**
Pure tone audiometry	ABR threshold evaluation
Extended high frequency audiometry	Tympanometry
Word recognition	
Tympanometry	

Monitoring: At risk patients will be evaluated weekly; high risk patients will be tested biweekly. The procedures will be as follows:

Alert Patients	**Non-Alert Patients**
Pure tone audiometry	ABR threshold evaluation
Extended high frequency audiometry	Tympanometry (when indicated)
Tympanometry (when indicated)	

Follow-up: Follow-up audiological evaluations will be conducted at 3 and 6 months after termination of ototoxic medications. Parents should be notified that the child is at risk for hearing impairment and follow-up evaluations will be recommended.

Ototoxic Medications: refer to Appendix A.

SUGGESTED SCHEDULE FOR MONITORING RENAL FUNCTION OF PATIENTS TREATED WITH AMINOGLYCOSIDES

1.   Patients with normal serum creatinine and
   a.   Treatment course of 14 days or less: determine serum creatinine at least twice weekly.
   b.   Treatment course of more than 14 days: determine serum creatinine at least three times at week.
2.   Patients with elevated but stable serum creatinine: determine serum creatinine at least every other day.
3.   Patients with rising or falling serum creatinine: determine serum creatinine at least once a day.

Source: Fairbanks, D. N. F. (1987). *Antimicrobial Therapy in Otolaryngology - Head and Neck Surgery.* Washington, D.C: The American Academy of Otolaryngology - Head and Neck Surgery Foundation.

SUGGESTED SCHEDULES FOR DETERMINATION OF AMINOGLYCOSIDE SERUM LEVELS

1.   Normal renal function
   a.   Peak level with first 1 to 2 days of therapy.
   b.   Trough level within 1 week.
   c.   Subsequently, peak and trough levels approximately once a week.
2   Impaired but stable renal function
   a.   Peak level within first 1 to 2 days of therapy.
   b.   Trough level and another peak level within 1 week.
   c.   Subsequently, peak and trough levels at least twice a week.
3.   Impaired but stable renal function
   a.   Peak and trough levels with first 1 to 2 days of therapy.
   b.   Determination of serum levels as often as daily thereafter for as long as renal function remains unstable.
4.   Following any adjustments of dosage, peak and trough levels should be determined within 1 to 2 days.
Peak serum levels are drawn 15 - 30 minutes after completion of an intravenous infusion or 60 minutes after an intramuscular injection. Trough levels are drawn 30 minutes before next dose.

Source: Fairbanks, D. N. F. (1987). *Antimicrobial Therapy in Otolaryngology - Head and Neck Surgery.* Washington, D.C: The American Academy of Otolaryngology - Head and Neck Surgery Foundations.

PRECAUTIONS FOR THE USE OF AMINOGLYCOSIDE THERAPY
IN PEDIATRIC PATIENTS

1.   To determine dosage, monitor serum aminoglycoside concentrations in infants with low birthweights and those with renal insufficiency.

2.   Higher than normal dosages may be necessary in children with cystic fibrosis and in some with malignancy. In patients with malignancies, serum concentrations should be measured to avoid toxic concentrations. Dosages should be on body surface rather than body weight.

3.   Avoid aminoglycoside therapy in patients receiving loop diuretics, indomethacin, or vancomycin and in patients with cholinergic dysfunction (e.g. myasthenia gravis or botulism).

4.   Monitor hearing and vestibular dysfunction in patients who receive prolonged therapy of high doses.

Source: McCraken, G. H. (1986). Aminoglycoside toxicity in infants and children. *The American Journal of Medicine, 80* (Supplement 6B), 172-178.

MEAN THRESHOLDS REFERENCED TO THE FLAT-PLATE COUPLER
(Stelmachowicz et. al. 1989[1], Hunter, 1993[2])

AGE	8	9	10	11	12	13	14	16	18	20 (kHz)
3-10[2]	18.2	21.5	20.5	24.0	29.0*	29.0*	33.2	45.4	64.8	86.4(dB SPL)
10-19[1]	14.4	19.8	20.9	22.4	27.1	33.1	37.7	58.1	74.2	95.8
20-29[1]	15.4	18.1	21.4	22.0	29.6	36.3	46.1	73.8	94.0	105.6
30-39[1]	17.2	20.7	24.4	26.2	34.3	41.0	49.9	87.5	106.1	111.3
40-49[1]	23.2	30.8	32.2	36.0	44.1	54.9	69.2	101.6	108.3	108.4
50-59[1]	44.9	52.6	62.1	67.5	81.1	91.5	105.0	122.4	124.3	121.4

*12.5 KHZ Thresholds from Hunter, 1993

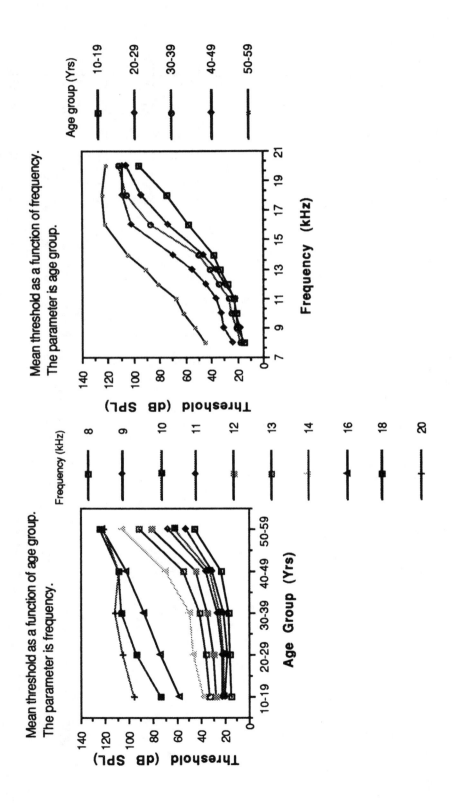

Mean threshold as a function of frequency.
The parameter is age group.

Mean threshold as a function of age group.
The parameter is frequency.

EXAMPLE OF AN EXTENDED HIGH FREQUENCY AUDIOGRAM

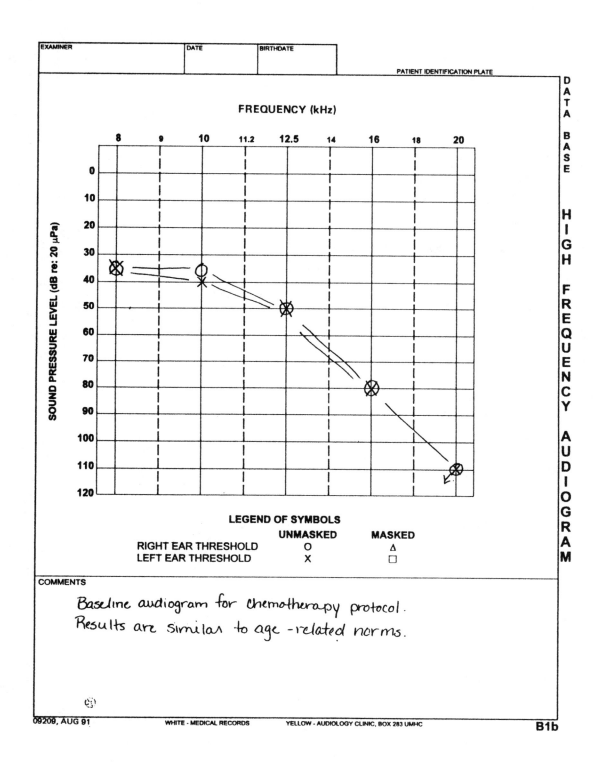

COMMENTS

Baseline audiogram for chemotherapy protocol.
Results are similar to age-related norms.

Section II Hearing Aid Evaluation, Fitting, & Follow Up

Protocol 7 Hearing Aid Consultation

Target Population: Any patient whose audiologic findings or personal complaints suggest possible benefit from amplification. Methods may need to be adapted for pediatric patients.

Rationale: The Hearing Aid Consultation is performed after the Basic Hearing Evaluation (Protocol 1). Its purpose is to a) educate the patient about amplification; b) obtain the necessary information to determine the patient's need for amplification; and, c) if needed, obtain the necessary information to write a hearing aid prescription.

Equipment Required:
Clinical audiometer with sound field capabilities
Real-ear measurement equipment
Hearing aid specification and matrix books

Methods:
1.   Determine the need for amplification from the results of the Basic Hearing Evaluation (Protocol 1) and by interviewing the patient regarding his/her acoustical, social, educational, and vocational environments; motivation; and acceptance of the hearing impairment. A weighing of all these factors will influence the decision.

2.   Counsel the patient about the benefits and limitations of hearing aids. Discuss the benefits of binaural amplification, when appropriate. Discuss the benefits of programmable hearing aids.

3.   Determine the type of hearing aid based on the patient's personal preference and physical dexterity, the degree and configuration of the hearing impairment, and interaural auditory differences.

4.   Determine which ear or ears to amplify based on the patient's acoustical, social, and vocational environments; auditory sensitivity; speech recognition; and financial resources. If speech recognition scores are depressed bilaterally (80% or below) or there is a 20% difference between scores on each ear, binaural speech recognition testing is completed to determine if binaural amplification will enhance word recognition ability. For binaural speech recognition testing, the input is 35 dB re: pure tone average for each ear, presented simultaneously to both ears. For sloping losses, a higher level may be necessary; this level should be 10 dB above the threshold at 3000 Hz.

5.   Determine the need for additional features such as a telecoil, pronounced volume control, audio input capabilities, etc., by discussing with the patient his/her listening environments and physical dexterity.

6.   Discuss options for obtaining a hearing aid. Provide information about the clinic hearing aid program (See Appendix F) and third party payments.

7.   Arrange for a signed medical authorization (authorization signatures must be no older than 6 months). If the patient is over 18 years old they may sign a waiver. (See Appendix E.) The patient should be encouraged to see the ENT physician if they have not done so in the past or if any changes have occurred in their hearing or otological health since the last ENT exam.

8.   Determine the patient's real-ear unaided response (REUR). Record the audiometric thresholds and the NAL calculation (Coupler Gain column) on lines one and two of the Hearing Aid Gain Worksheet (HAGW -- see Appendix B). Perform the real-ear unaided response measurement. Enter the values in the right hand column as the REUR in line three of the HAGW.

9.   If a conductive loss is present add the air-bone gap as the Conductive Correction on line 5 of the HAGW. If a bone conduction threshold cannot be obtained at the limits of the audiometer, it will be estimated.

10.   Determine the required 2cc coupler full-on-gain (F.O.G.) by adding the columns in the HAGW. Note that an experienced hearing aid user may want more gain than the NAL formulae suggest.

11.   Determine maximum acoustic output (SSPL90). The SSPL90 should be sufficiently low so amplified sound does not become uncomfortably loud when the volume wheel is set for speech at comfortable levels. For average adult hearing losses less than 70 dB the peak SSPL90 should not be greater than 115 dB SPL, with a range of 105 to 115. For losses of 70 to 80 dB add 5 dB; for 85 to 90 dB losses add 10 dB; and for losses greater than 95 dB add 15 dB. These values should be decreased by 10 dB for infants and by 5 dB for young children.

12.   Use the information obtained above to write a prescription, as appropriate. Custom ITE electroacoustic specifications can either be chosen by matching specifications provided in matrix books, or alternatively, F.O.G. and SSPL can be specified for inclusion on the order form. *Manufacturers will often choose to meet only circuit specifications if you supply them, disregarding your specified F.O.G.* Prescribe frequency and output trimmers whenever possible.

13.   When prescribing amplification for young children, additional considerations must be made: flexibility of controls as the audiogram may not be fully defined; size of the unit; audio input and electromagnetic pickup capabilities; use of a battery compartment door lock and/or volume control cover; the purchase of additional loss and damage coverage; financial assistance; and educational/rehabilitation follow-up services for long term hearing aid orientation/evaluation.

Report Format:
A brief note is written into the patient's chart by the dated "Audiology Clinic" stamp in the "Outpatient progress notes" section. See Appendices A through E for the following forms: Hearing Aid Consultation, Hearing Aid Prescription, Hearing Aid Gain Worksheet, and Medical Release and Waiver Forms. The following forms are filed reverse-chronologically in the patient's dispensing chart: Hearing Aid Consultation Checklist, Gain Worksheet, Medical Release Form, Probe Measurement Results, Basic Hearing Evaluation Results, Progress Notes, ENT Notes (if appropriate), Patient Questionnaires. A copy of the patient's hospital chart face sheet

is placed in the back of the dispensing chart. If the patient will be obtaining the hearing aid outside the program, the patient is given the original Medical Release Form and Hearing Aid Prescription (copies of which are placed in the dispensing chart), as well as a copy of the Audiology Record Form (see Protocol 1).

Billing:
Bill one unit of Hearing Rehabilitation (CPT 92507) for each 15-minute block of time or one unit of Consultation (CPT 99242) for each 10-minute block of time. If the patient will be obtaining the hearing aid outside this facility, charge one unit of Hearing Aid Consultation (CPT 92590) for each 30-minute block of time. Charge the appropriate Clinic Visit fee for all patients.

References:

Byrne, D., & Dillon, H. (1986). Hearing aids and aural rehabilitation: The National Acoustic Laboratories' (NAL) new procedure for selecting the gain and frequency response of a hearing aid. *Ear and Hearing, 7*, 257-265.

Lybarger, S. F., & Teder, H. (1986). 2cc coupler curves to insertion gain curves: Calculated and experimental results. *Hearing Instruments, 37*, 36-40.

Matkin, N. D. (1981). Hearing aids for children. In W. R. Hodgson & P. H. Skinner (Eds.), *Hearing Aid Assessment and Use in Audiologic Habilitation* (pp. 171-195). Baltimore, MD: Williams & Wilkins.

Mueller, H., Hawkins, D., & Northern, J. (1992). *Probe Microphone Measurements: Hearing Aid Selection and Assessment.* San Diego: Singular Publishing Group, Inc.

Mueller, H. G., & Killion, M. C. (1990). An easy method for calculating the articulation index. *The Hearing Journal, 43*, 14-17.

Pascoe, D. P. (1985). Hearing aid evaluation. In J. Katz (Ed.), *Handbook of Clinical Audiology* (pp. 936-948). Baltimore: Williams & Wilkins.

Pavlovic, C. V. (1989). Speech spectrum considerations and speech intelligibility predictions in hearing aid evaluations. *Journal of Speech and Hearing Disorders, 54*, 3-8.

Pavlovic, C. V. (1991). Speech recognition and five articulation indexes. *Hearing Instruments, 42*, 20-23.

Skinner, M. W. (1988). *Hearing Aid Evaluation.* Englewood Cliffs: Prentice Hall.

Skinner, P. H. (1981). Relationship of electro-and psychoacoustic measures. In W. R. Hodgson & P. H. Skinner (Eds.), *Hearing Aid Assessment and Use in Audiologic Habilitation* (pp. 131-151). Baltimore: Williams & Wilkins.

Valente, M. (1994). *Strategies for Selecting and Verifying Hearing Aid Fittings.* New York: Thieme Medical Publishers, Inc.

Protocol 7 Appendix

A.   Hearing Aid Consultation Checklist
B.   Hearing Aid Gain Worksheet
C.   Hearing Aid Prescription
D.   Food And Drug Administration Regulation Concerning The Sale Of Hearing Aids
E.   Waiver Of Medical Evaluation
F.   Hearing Aid Program

HEARING AID CONSULTATION CHECKLIST

Patient Name: _____   Date: _____
Hosp. Number: _____

_____ Listening Environment _____
_____
_____

_____ Assessment of Amplification Needs
Audiologist's Impressions: _____
Patient's Impressions: _____
_____ Hearing Aid Benefits and Limitations_____
_____

_____ Binaural/Monaural   _____
_____

_____ Programmable/Conventional _____
_____

_____ Style of Hearing Aid_____
_____

_____ Telephone Use (telecoil)_____
_____

_____ Outside Activities (wind screen) _____
_____

_____ Physical Dexterity (pronounced VC, removal notches) _____
_____

_____ Assistive Listening Devices (audio input and telecoil) _____
_____

_____ Hearing Aid Recommended _____Yes _____ No   _____
_____

_____ Third Party Payment _ _____
_____

_____ Where to get Hearing Aids_____
_____

_____ Medical Release_____
_____

_____ Prediction of Success_____
_____

_____ Comments_____
_____

_____
Audiologist

HEARING AID GAIN WORKSHEET

Audiologist	Date

RIGHT EAR

	250	500	750	1000	1500	2000	3000	4000	6000
Audiometric Thresholds (Date of test_____)....									
NAL-R 2cc F.O.G....................									
REUR..................................	+	+	+	+	+	+	+	+	+
Kemar Response...................	- 0	- 1	- 1	- 2	- 3	- 9	- 15	- 12	- 5
Conductive Correction (.5 x air-bone gap).................	+	+	+	+	+	+	+	+	+
Required 2cc F.O.G........									
1 Date_____Delivered F.O.G.									
Delivered minus Required F.O.G.									
2 Date_____Delivered F.O.G.									
Delivered minus Required F.O.G.									

Required REIR.............									
Date_____Measured REIR									
Measured minus Required REIR									

LEFT EAR

	250	500	750	1000	1500	2000	3000	4000	6000
Audiometric Thresholds (Date of test_____)....									
NAL-R 2cc F.O.G....................									
REUR..................................	+	+	+	+	+	+	+	+	+
Kemar Response...................	- 0	- 1	- 1	- 2	- 3	- 9	- 15	- 12	- 5
Conductive Correction (.5 x air-bone gap).................	+	+	+	+	+	+	+	+	+
Required 2cc F.O.G........									
1 Date_____Delivered F.O.G.									
Delivered minus Required F.O.G.									
2 Date_____Delivered F.O.G.									
Delivered minus Required F.O.G.									

Required REIR.............									
Date_____Measured REIR									
Measured minus Required REIR									

HEARING AID PRESCRIPTION

NAME _____ UH#_____ DATE_____

BTE:

MANUFACTURER & MODEL _____

Ear: R _____ L _____ Bin. _____   Battery: _____

OPTIONS: SETTINGS:

Hook _____ Color _____ Tone _____ Output _____ Gain _____ AGC _____

REMARKS: _____

EARMOLD:

MANUFACTURER _____ R _____ L _____ Bin. _____

STYLE: MATERIAL: LOSS:

_____ Shell/Full Shell   _____ Lucite   _____ Mild

_____ Half Shell   _____ Silicone   _____ Moderate

_____ Phantom/Skeleton   _____ Polyethylene (Hypoallergenic) _____ Severe

_____ Half Phantom/Half Skeleton _____ Formaseal   _____ Profound

_____ Canal   _____ Other

_____ CROS   MISCELLANEOUS: EAR TEXTURE:

TUBING: _____ Select-A-Vent   _____ Soft

_____ Size   _____ Sound Separator   _____ Medium

_____ Horn (3mm or 4mm)   _____ Color _____   _____ Firm

_____ Other _____   _____ Other _____

REMARKS: _____

ITE:

MANUFACTURER & MODEL _____

Ear: R _____ L _____ Bin. _____   Color: _____   Battery: _____

CIRCUIT SPECIFICATION:

      250   500   750   1000   1500   2000   3000   4000Hz

R-2cc FOG   _____dB SPL Matrix _____

L-2cc FOG   _____dB SPL Matrix _____

COST OPTIONS: NO-COST OPTIONS:

_____ Tone (low freq) Control _____   _____ Windscreen (Hood or Screen)

_____ Output Limiter _____   _____ Removal Notches

_____ Feedback (high freq) Limiter _____ _____ Built-Up Volume Control

_____ Telecoil _____   _____ Canal Length _____

_____ On-Off Switch _____   _____ Wax Guard _____ Extd Rcvr Tube

_____ Class D Receiver _____   _____ Selector-Switch Style

_____ Compression: ____K-Amp ____Adap Comp   Venting: _____No Vent _____Pressure

                     ____other_____   _____SAV (specify size)

                     _____ IROS (full or adjustable)

REMARKS: _____

MEDICAL RELEASE: _____ ,M.D.

AUDIOLOGIST: _____

This prescription is valid for a maximum period of six months from above date, or less if there is a
significant change in hearing. After six months, further evaluation would be required prior to obtaining
a hearing aid. THIS PRESCRIPTION OR RECOMMENDATION MAY BE FILLED BY, AND HEARING
INSTRUMENTS MAY BE PURCHASED FROM, THE CERTIFIED DISPENSER OF YOUR CHOICE.

FOOD AND DRUG ADMINISTRATION REGULATION
CONCERNING THE SALE OF HEARING AIDS

On August 25, 1977, the Food and Drug Administration (FDA) regulation concerning the sale of hearing aids became effective. The regulation requires individuals with a hearing loss to have a medical evaluation by a licensed physician (preferably a physician specializing in diseases of the ear) within six (6) months preceding the purchase of a hearing aid.

Fully informed adults may request that the medical evaluation be waived for personal or religious reasons. The medical evaluation is mandatory for persons under eighteen (18) years of age.

The physician should provide the patient with a written statement indicating that the patient's hearing loss has been medically evaluated and that there are no medical contraindications for hearing aid use. The statement should be presented to the hearing aid dispenser prior to purchasing the instrument.

_____ was examined by me on

_____, 19___. My examination did not reveal any medical

conditions which would contraindicate hearing aid use.

_____
Physician's Signature

_____
(Typed or Printed)

_____
Address

_____
City   State   Zip Code

_____
Phone Number

WAIVER OF MEDICAL EVALUATION

I have been advised by the dispenser from the University, that the Food and Drug Administration has determined that my best interest would be served if I had a medical evaluation by a licensed physician (preferably a physician who specializes in diseases of the ear) before purchasing a hearing aid.

I do not wish a medical evaluation before purchasing a hearing aid.

_____   _____

Signature   Date

HEARING AID PROGRAM

Patients who obtain hearing aids through this facility participate in a 1-year program that is designed to insure that an appropriate hearing aid is selected, that it is fit properly to the patient's ear, and that the hearing aid user is properly instructed in the care and use of the device. The following is a description of the program.

1. **Medical Consultation.** Each patient who is evaluated for a hearing aid is encouraged to see a physician to rule out medical treatment for the hearing disorder.

2. **Hearing Evaluation.** The first step in the hearing aid program is to obtain a thorough evaluation of the patient's hearing. The evaluation may differ among patients, but includes hearing tests that employ tones and speech. A test of middle ear function is usually obtained as well. If the patient has not been examined by a physician, this should be done before the next step.

3. **Hearing Aid Consultation.** The patient will receive information regarding the types of hearing aids that are appropriate for his/her hearing loss. A prescription will be written containing the characteristics of the appropriate hearing aid. The prescription can be filled by any certified hearing aid dispenser. If the patient chooses to obtain the hearing aid from this facility, an impression of the ear will be taken and the hearing aid will be ordered. A deposit is due at the time the order is placed. When the hearing aid is received, it will be tested to insure that it is working properly.

4. **Hearing Aid Fitting.** The patient will return and the hearing aid will be fit to the patient's ear. Listening tests will be conducted to determine that the hearing aid is functioning effectively. The patient will receive instruction on the care and use of the hearing aid. It is often helpful if other family members are present during this instruction. The balance of the charges for the hearing aid is due at the time of the hearing aid fitting.

5. **Initial Review.** Between two and four weeks after the fitting, the patient will return for a check of the hearing aid. Again, tests will be conducted to determine the effectiveness of the hearing aid. The patient should write down any problems that he/she experiences with the hearing aid and discuss these with the audiologist at the initial review. The hearing aid may be adjusted at this time. If the patient is not satisfied with the hearing aid, it can be returned for a refund (less a service fee). There is no additional charge for the initial review.

6. **Hearing Aid Orientation.** The patient is invited to participate in a group hearing aid orientation session. Two or three hearing aid users and their family members typically participate in these sessions. The group session provides the patient an opportunity to discuss his/her experiences and concerns with other hearing aid users, gives family members some understanding of hearing impairment, and includes a discussion of strategies for better listening. There is no additional charge for this session.

7. **Annual Review.** Before the end of the first year the patient will return for a hearing test and hearing aid check. Again, tests will be performed to measure the effectiveness of the hearing aid. If adjustments are necessary, they will be made at the annual review. There is no additional charge for the annual review of the hearing aid.

HEARING AID PROGRAM *page 2*

Any problems related to the hearing aid will be addressed without additional charge during the year that begins with the hearing aid fitting. This does not include fees for test procedures not related to the hearing aid.

Protocol 8 Hearing-Aid Fitting (HAF)

Target Population:
Patients who have ordered hearing aids through this facility.

Rationale:
The Hearing-Aid Fitting is performed a) to insure that the recommended hearing aid(s) meet(s) the specifications of the prescribing audiologist; b) to instruct the patient on hearing-aid use and care; and c) to verify that the recommended hearing aid is performing adequately on the patient.

Equipment Required:
Electroacoustic hearing-aid analyzer with real-ear measurement capabilities
Clinical audiometer with soundfield capabilities
Telephone
Programmable hearing-instrument equipment

Methods:
1.   Prior to the HAF, the hearing aid should be checked.
      a.   Physical Features. The recommended features (e.g. raised volume control, venting, trimmers, filters, etc.) should be present.
      b.   Listening Check. The hearing aid should be checked for intermittency, distortion, volume-control taper, noise, telecoil function, and on/off switch operation.
      c.   Mechanical Check. The physical components of the hearing aid, such as the battery compartment, trimmers, and switches should be manipulated.
      d.   Electroacoustic Check. Refer To Protocol 9 Electroacoustic Hearing-Aid Evaluation.
      If problems are noted, the hearing aid should be returned to the manufacturer for repair or replacement.

2.   Perform clinical assessment of hearing-aid gain. Obtain real-ear measurements.   If there are problems obtaining real-ear measures due to feedback before use gain, patient report of discomfort, difficulty placing the probe tube, or lack of patient cooperation, functional-gain measures should be obtained.
      a.   Real-Ear Insertion Gain: Using a real-ear measurement system, select the desired target insertion-gain response (e.g. NAL-R, POGO, Custom). For cases of conductive or mixed hearing loss, enter the bone-conduction thresholds, instead of air-conduction thresholds, for calculating the target gain, and add the air-bone gap to the calculated target-gain values. Estimate the bone-conduction thresholds if they exceed the limits of the audiometer. After the target gain has been calculated, seat the patient, position the speaker, place the probe tube, and level the instrument as instructed in Appendix A. Obtain the real-ear unaided response (REUR). Insert the hearing aid or

earmold, adjust the volume control to approximately 50% of full rotation, and obtain the real-ear insertion response (REIR), using a 65 dB SPL composite noise. Repeat the REIR while adjusting the trimpots to yield a response which matches the target gain. Turn the volume to the full-on position or slightly below the feedback point and obtain a final REIR to insure 10-15 dB of reserve gain.

Using the REIR gain measurements and unaided thresholds, aided thresholds should be estimated. The goal is to maximize the audibility of the speech spectrum, which can be approximated by the area of the aided audiogram between 20 and 50 dB HL, 500-4000 Hz. If the estimated aided thresholds do not indicate adequate gain, further modifications are indicated. These include adjusting the trimmers, modifying the earmold or hearing-aid shell, reprogramming, and/or sending the hearing aid to the manufacturer for circuit changes, recasing, or replacement.

b.   Functional Gain. Seat the patient at 45 degrees azimuth relative to the loudspeaker. Instruct the patient to adjust the gain control so that the recorded Rainbow Passage presented at 40 dB HL (conversational level speech) is comfortably loud and clearly intelligible. If probe-microphone measures were completed, set the volume control and trimmers to the settings at which the REIR best matched the target gain. Obtain unaided and aided soundfield thresholds (functional gain), plugging or masking the non-test ear, if necessary. Record the settings and volume control rotation on the aided audiogram. There should be 10-15 dB reserve gain above the comfort setting. If the aided audiogram does not indicate adequate audibility of the speech spectrum, modifications are indicated. These include adjusting the trimmers, modifying the earmold or hearing-aid shell, counseling the patient on setting the volume control, reprogramming, and/or sending the hearing aid to the manufacturer for circuit changes, recasing, or replacement.

3.   Perform clinical assessment of aided uncomfortable loudness levels (UCL). Again, use real-ear measures unless problems, as indicated previously, preclude its use:

a.   Real-Ear Aided UCL Check. Following REIR measurements, set the volume to the full-on position or slightly below the feedback point. The output limiter should be adjusted to the highest setting that corresponds closest to measured loudness-discomfort levels. Obtain the real-ear saturation response (RESR), using a 90 dB SPL sweep-frequency tone, to document the maximum tolerable real-ear output of the aid and to assess whether the peak SSPL90 value exceeds the maximum value specified in Step 11 of Protocol 4.5. If when the output trimmer is set to the minimum output and discomfort persists, the hearing aid may need to be changed or sent to the manufacturer for circuit changes.

b.   Soundfield Aided UCL Check. To check SSPL90, use the procedure recommended by Beattie (1988) and Skinner (1988)using a 90 dB SPL complex or speech stimulus. The patient should be seated at 45 degrees azimuth relative to the loudspeaker. The output should be adjusted to the highest setting at which the patient tolerates 90 dB SPL of speech noise for 10 seconds, while wearing the hearing aid at full-on or just below feedback. If uncomfortable, decrease the output and repeat the procedure. If when the output trimmer is set to the minimum output, and discomfort persists, the hearing aid may need to be changed or sent to the manufacturer for circuit changes.

4.   Modify earmold or custom hearing-aid shell if necessary, as indicated by the patient's complaints of discomfort, hollow quality, feedback, etc. Repeat real-ear or functional-gain testing as warranted.

5.   Provide information for the following areas as outlined on the Hearing-Aid Fitting Form (see Appendix B): hearing-aid use, care, and storage; varied listening situations; expectations; troubleshooting; wind noise; moisture; cerumen management, assistive-listening devices; battery use, storage/disposal, and associated health hazards. The Safety Rules and Warning Form (see Appendix C) should be read and signed by the patient.

6.   Provide information, demonstration, and practice on hearing aid/earmold insertion and removal, volume-control adjustment, battery insertion and removal, hearing aid and earmold cleaning, trouble shooting, daily maintenance, and telephone use. The patient should be given the opportunity to try their hearing aid with the telephone (using either a taped message or calls from another phone) and accompanying telephone listening devices.

Report Format:
Insert the original Hearing-Aid Fitting Form in the medical record and a copy in the hearing-aid dispensing chart. Also included in the dispensing chart are the following: electroacoustic results; soundfield aided/unaided or real-ear measurement results, and; signed copy of the Safety Rules and Warning statement.

Billing:
No charge.

References:
Beattie, R. C. (1988). SSPL selection -- A clinical protocol. *The Hearing Journal, 41,* 18-22.

Byrne, D., & Dillon, H. (1986). The National Acoustic Laboratories' (NAL) new procedure for selecting the gain and frequency response of a hearing aid. *Ear and Hearing, 7,* 257-265.

Hawkins, D. B. (1987). Clinical ear canal probe tube measurements. *Ear and Hearing, 8,* 74S-81S.

Hawkins, D. B., & H. G. Mueller (1986). Some variables affecting the accuracy of probe tube microphone measurements. *Hearing Instruments, 37,* 8-12, 49.

Killion, M. C., & Revit, L. J. (1987). Insertion gain repeatability versus loudspeaker location: You want me to put my loudspeaker WHERE?' *Ear and Hearing, 8,* 68S-73S.

Mueller, H., Hawkins, D., & Northern, J. (1992). *Probe Microphone Measurements: Hearing Aid Selection and Assessment.* San Diego: Singular Publishing Group, Inc.

Skinner, M. W. (1988). *Hearing Aid Evaluation.* Englewood Cliffs: Prentice Hall.

Valente, M. (1994). *Strategies for Selecting and Verifying Hearing Aid Fittings.* New York: Thieme Medical Publishers, Inc.

Protocol 7 Appendix

A.   Real-Ear Measurement Set-Up
B.   Hearing Aid Fitting Checklist
C.   Hearing Aid Safety Rules and Warnings
D.   Special Announcement to All Hearing-Aid Dispensary Patients

REAL-EAR MEASUREMENT SET-UP

I.   Positioning the patient and speaker:

1.   Position the speaker approximately 12 inches from the patient's head towards the ear to be tested.

2.   Adjust the angle of the speaker to an azimuth of 45 degrees , approximately halfway between the patient's nose and ear, and 45 degrees above the level of the ear.

II.   Placement of the probe tube:

1.   Clean the probe tube and ear hook with an alcohol wipe. Allow to dry for one minute.

2.   Mark the tube using a constant length of 30 mm.

3.   Place the Velcro headband on the patient's head above the ears and attach the reference microphone, facing forward, directly above the ear to be tested.

4.   Attach the body of the probe microphone on the ear hanger.

5.   Place the probe tube (without the earmold or aid) into the ear until the 30 mm mark is at the tragal notch.

III.   Leveling the real-ear measurement system:

1.   Position the speaker, reference microphone, and probe tube, as described in this Appendix sections I and II, and level.

2.   If the leveling process is unsuccessful, check the following: (a) position of the speaker; (b) connection of the microphone to the measurement system, (c) cerumen in the probe tube and/or (d) calibration of the soundfield speaker and the microphones (refer to the equipment manual for instruction).

HEARING AID FITTING CHECKLIST

DATE					Output Clinic Notes
AID/S	RIGHT/MANUFACTURER	SERIAL NO.	PATIENT IDENTIFICATION PLATE		
	LEFT/MANUFACTURER	SERIAL NO.			
	REMOTE CONTROL MODEL	SERIAL NO.			

	CHECKLIST	**COMMENTS**	
☐	Hearing Aid Settings		**H**
☐	Modification of Earmold/Shell		**E**
☐	Functional Gain		**A**
☐	Real-Ear Measurements		**R**
☐	**PATIENT INSTRUCTION**		**I**
☐	Inserting Aid/Earmold		**N**
☐	Adjusting Volume/Switches/Remote Control		**G**
☐	Battery Insertion/Drain/Warning Signal		
☐	Cleaning Aid/Earmold		**A**
☐	Telephone Use/Pads/Amplifiers		**I**
☐	Difficult Listening Situations		**D**
☐	Initial Use Schedule		
☐	Expectations		**F**
☐	Trouble-Shooting (wax & battery)		**I**
☐	Servicing/Warranty (Clinic & Manufacturer)/Loss Coverage		**T**
☐	When not to Wear Aid		**T**
☐	Moisture/Consequent Problems/Dri-Aid Kit		**I**
☐	Storage (away from pets & children)		**N**
☐	Health Hazards of Batteries		**G**
☐	Assistive Listening Devices		
☐	Cerumen Management/Wax Guards		
☐	Other		
☐	Return Appointment		
		Audiologist	

HEARING AID SAFETY RULES AND WARNINGS

HEARING AIDS AND BATTERIES CAN BE DANGEROUS IF IMPROPERLY USED OR SWALLOWED AND CAN RESULT IN SEVERE INJURY, PERMANENT HEARING LOSS, OR DEATH.

• Hearing aids should be used only as directed and adjusted by your audiologist. Misuse can result in sudden and permanent hearing loss.

• Never allow others to wear your hearing aid. Misused hearing aids can permanently damage another's hearing.

• Hearing aids may stop functioning without warning, for instance when the battery goes dead. You should be aware of this possibility, particularly when circulating in traffic or otherwise depending on warning sounds.

• Hearing aids, parts, accessories, and batteries are not toys and should be kept out of reach of anyone who might swallow these items or otherwise cause themselves injury.

• Never change the battery or adjust the controls of the hearing aid in the presence of infants, small children, or persons of mental incapacity.

• Always check medication before swallowing. Batteries can be mistaken for tablets.

• Never put your hearing aid or batteries in your mouth for any reason. Hearing aids and batteries are slippery and may be swallowed.

• Do not store loose batteries in your pockets. Batteries that touch each other can cause an electrical current that could burn you.

• Recycle used batteries by returning them to your hearing aid dispenser or depositing them at a Button Battery Collection Box located at Target, Snyder's Drug Store, or Black's Photography. Otherwise, discard batteries carefully in a place where they cannot be reached by infants, small children, or persons of mental incapacity.

In the event hearing aid batteries are swallowed, **see a doctor immediately** and call the
NATIONAL BUTTON BATTERY HOTLINE, collect **(202)625-3333**.

I have read and understand the above "Hearing Aid Safety Rules and Warnings."

Signature_____   Date_____

Audiologist_____   Date_____

HEARING AID SAFETY RULES AND WARNINGS

HEARING AIDS AND BATTERIES CAN BE DANGEROUS IF IMPROPERLY USED OR SWALLOWED AND CAN RESULT IN SEVERE INJURY, PERMANENT HEARING LOSS, OR DEATH.

- Hearing aids should be used only as directed and adjusted by your audiologist. Misuse can result in sudden and permanent hearing loss.

- Never allow others to wear your hearing aid. Misused hearing aids can permanently damage another's hearing.

- Hearing aids may stop functioning without warning, for instance when the battery goes dead. You should be aware of this possibility, particularly when circulating in traffic or otherwise depending on warning sounds.

- Hearing aids, parts, accessories, and batteries are not toys and should be kept out of reach of anyone who might swallow these items or otherwise cause themselves injury.

- Never change the battery or adjust the controls of the hearing aid in the presence of infants, small children, or persons of mental incapacity.

- Always check medication before swallowing. Batteries can be mistaken for tablets.

- Never put your hearing aid or batteries in your mouth for any reason. Hearing aids and batteries are slippery and may be swallowed.

- Do not store loose batteries in your pockets. Batteries that touch each other can cause an electrical current that could burn you.

- Recycle used batteries by returning them to your hearing aid dispenser or depositing them at a Button Battery Collection Box located at Target, Snyder's Drug Store, or Black's Photography. Otherwise, discard batteries carefully in a place where they cannot be reached by infants, small children, or persons of mental incapacity.

In the event hearing aid batteries are swallowed, **see a doctor immediately** and call the
NATIONAL BUTTON BATTERY HOTLINE, collect **(202)625-3333**.

I have read and understand the above "Hearing Aid Safety Rules and Warnings."

Signature_____   Date_____

Audiologist_____   Date_____

SPECIAL ANNOUNCEMENT

TO ALL HEARING-AID DISPENSARY PATIENTS

On _____ 19_____

From _____ to _____

This clinic will offer a hearing-aid orientation and rehabilitation program for new hearing-aid users. We encourage and welcome close family members or friends to attend with you.

OBJECTIVES:

1.   To review hearing-aid use, care, maintenance, and problem solving.

2.   To provide information about hearing loss and associated problems.

3.   To provide tips to improve listening skills.

4.   To let family members and friends experience what it is like to have a hearing loss.

COST: Free to all hearing-aid dispensary patient's. This program is part of the comprehensive hearing-health care provided at this clinic. We offer this service as an extension of our hearing-aid dispensing program.

REGISTER: with our receptionist or call 555-5775. If your call is long distance, please use our toll-free number, 1-800-555-5252.

Protocol 9 Initial (Hearing Aid) Review

Target population:
The Initial Review is performed before the end of the 30 day trial period following the hearing aid fitting.

Rationale:
The purpose of the Initial Review is: a) to ensure that the hearing aid continues to function to specifications; b) to verify that the patient is using amplification devices effectively; c) to adjust hearing aid parameters as needed; d) to continue to educate the patient regarding hearing, hearing loss and hearing aid use; e) to prepare the hearing aid user to be self sufficient in managing the amplification device.

Equipment required:
Electroacoustic hearing aid analyzer with Real ear capabilities
Battery tester
Telephone
Screwdriver
Wax loop and brush
Grinding and buffing tools
Magnifying glass

Methods:
Hearing aids will be evaluated following the Initial Review Checklist provided in Appendix A.

1. Subjective Evaluation. The audiologist explores the quality of the patient's experience with the hearing aid(s). Among the considerations should be: physical fit, word clarity, sound quality, loudness, occlusion effect (be aware that if this effect is only noted with the user's own voice and not others, a final remedy may be a significant lengthening of the canal), feedback, internal noise, speech recognition in noise and groups, radio and television, telephone/telephone coil, male vs. female and children's voices, binaural/monaural impressions, important occasions and other issues.

2. Use Schedule/Battery Life. The patient will report their hearing aid usage schedule for each ear. The record of battery life should be consistent with the use schedule and expected battery drain.

3. Mechanical Function.
a) The audiologist will confirm that the patient can easily insert and remove the instrument. The patient should demonstrate adequate hand coordination and manipulation of instrument.
b) The patient should demonstrate proper battery insertion and removal.
c) The audiologist will review techniques for telephone use including use of a telecoil, telephone

receiver pads, and telephone amplifiers.

4. Volume Control Use. The patient will demonstrate proper manipulation of the volume control. The audiologist will report the volume control use position and the position when feedback occurs.

5. Removal/Storage/Cleaning. The patient will demonstrate the proper removal of the instrument, opening of battery drawer, storage, and discuss hearing aid dehumidifiers. The patient will demonstrate wax removal procedures with wax loop and/or brush.

6. Conventional/Programmable Settings. The audiologist will document the settings for each aid as determined at the time of the hearing aid fitting and any changes made at the time at the Initial Review. A careful record should be kept of any change in the original prescription.

7. Physical Modification. A physical modification may be necessary which includes grinding and buffing for a more comfortable fit in the ear, vent enlargement for modification of frequency response or control of occlusion effect. Document any modifications.

8. Testing.
a) Electroacoustic Check: The hearing aid should be checked electroacoustically at use and/or full-on gain settings. Refer to Protocol 12 Electroacoustic Hearing Aid Evaluation.

b) Functional Gain or Real Ear Insertion Response (REIR): Functional gain or REIR should be measured if significant physical modifications are made in the hearing aid or if settings are changed.

9. Continued Usage. The patient's interest to continue usage should be recorded for each hearing aid.

10. Return Appointment. Most adults will return in eleven months. Earlier appointments should be made when independent usage has not been demonstrated or when additional fine tuning is required.

Report Format:

Initial Review Checklist placed in Dispensing Chart (Refer to Appendix A)
Electroacoustic results placed in Dispensing Chart
Notation made in hospital chart.

Billing:

No charge if the hearing aid was purchased from your clinic's hearing aid dispensary. If the aid was purchased elsewhere the appropriate number of consultation units will be charged for the time spent with the patient and a clinic visit fee.

References:

Hodgson, W.R. (1981). Learning hearing aid use. In W.R. Hodgson and P.H. Skinner (Ed.), Hearing aid assessment and use in audiologic habilitation. Baltimore: Williams & Wilkins, pp. 212-225.

Loavenbruck, A.M. ; Madell, J.F. (1981). Hearing aid dispensing for audiologists. New York: Grune & Stratton.

Sandlin, R.E. (1994). Understanding digitally programmable hearing aids. Needham Heights, MA: Allyn and Bacon.

Skinner, M.W. (1988). Hearing aid evaluation. Englewood Cliffs, N.J.: Prentice Hall.

Protocol 9 Appendix

A.   Initial Review Checklist

INITIAL REVIEW CHECKLIST

Examiner	Date	Birthdate

	Manufacturer	Model	Serial Number
R			
L			
Rem Ctrl			

Subjective Evaluation

- ☐ Physical Fit _____
- ☐ Word Clarity _____
- ☐ Sound Quality _____
- ☐ Loudness _____
- ☐ Occlusion Effect _____
- ☐ Feedback _____
- ☐ Internal Noise _____
- ☐ Background Noise _____
- ☐ Groups _____
- ☐ Radio and T.V. _____
- ☐ Telephone/Telecoil _____
- ☐ Male vs. Female _____
- ☐ Monaural vs Binaural _____
- ☐ Problem Situations _____
- ☐ Other _____

_____
_____
_____
_____
_____
_____
_____

Use Schedule/Battery Life

	Curr Dr (mA)	Exp. Hrs/day	Act. Hrs/day
R			
L			

Mechanical Function (Patient Demo)

- ☐ Insertion of Instrument _____
- ☐ Removal _____
- ☐ Insertion of Battery _____
- ☐ Removal _____
- ☐ Motor Skills _____
- ☐ Telephone Practice _____

Volume Control Use

- ☐ Speed, ease _____
- ☐ MCL Position _____
- ☐ Feedback Point _____

Removal/Storage/Cleaning

- ☐ Removal/Storage _____
- ☐ Dri-Aid Kit _____
- ☐ Wax Removal _____
- ☐ Wax Guard System _____

Conventional Settings

Initial ◯ ◯ ◯ ◯ ◯ ◯
         ___ ___ ___ ___ ___ ___

Final   ◯ ◯ ◯ ◯ ◯ ◯
         ___ ___ ___ ___ ___ ___

Programmable Settings

Initial _____
        _____
Final   _____
        _____

Physical Modification

- ☐ Shell _____
- ☐ Earmold _____
- ☐ Other (vent/tonehook) _____

Testing

- ☐ Electroacoustics _____
- ☐ Functional Gain _____
- ☐ Real Ear _____

Continued Usage

    Yes No   Yes No
R ☐ ☐ L ☐ ☐

Return Appt. ☐3 ☐6 ☐9 ☐11 Months

Comments/Recommendations _____
_____
_____
_____
_____
_____
_____
_____
_____
_____
_____
_____

Protocol 10 **Hearing-Aid Orientation**

Target Population:
Hearing-aid users, family members, and friends.

Rationale:
Provide an informal group session to: a) review hearing-aid use and care; and, b) discuss hearing impairment and associated communication problems with family members and friends. The session should be attended after a few weeks of hearing-aid use and can be scheduled on the same date as the initial hearing-aid review. An information sheet is given to the patients at the time of the hearing aid fitting. Discussions are encouraged during the session to maintain the informal atmosphere.

Equipment Required:
Tape recorder
Slide projector
Paper and pencils
Handouts on organizations supporting people with hearing impairment

Methods:
Present information on the following:

1. _Auditory System_. Slides are used to describe the auditory system and transmission of sound. This information is related to causes and types of hearing impairment.

2. _Hearing-Aid Function_. The major components of hearing aids are described. Slides in this section show the different styles of hearing aids and introduce some of the inherent limitations such as amplification of background noise and poor communicative situations.

3. _Hearing-Aid Problems and Difficult Listening Situations_. Problems and situations are discussed and related to the user's own experiences. These include background noise, wind, feedback, patient's voice, fullness, telephone use, TV viewing, listening at church/temple, lectures, meetings, groups, and movies. Appropriate assistive listening devices (ALDs) are included in this discussion. Participants are encouraged to refer back to their prescribing audiologist for more details on ALDs if they are encountering problems. Some examples of the ALDs discussed are:

> Telephone--amplifiers attached to their phone, relay service and speakers
> Television--infra-red systems, closed captioning, direct input connections, and induction coil systems.
> Church/Temple/Auditorium--infra-red systems, induction coil systems, listings of places with amplifier (see references).
> Groups/Meetings--individualized audio-input systems and personal headsets.

4.   Daily Hearing-Aid Care. Users are asked to provide information on how they care for their hearing aid at the end and beginning of the day. Responses and/or suggestions should include opening the battery compartment, cleaning the hearing aid (wiping the case with a dry cloth) and/or earmold, and removing wax from the ITE receiver port or earmold sound bore. Also included are keeping batteries and hearing aids away from children and pets.

5.   Trouble Shooting Hearing-Aid Problems. Users are asked to give solutions they would try if their hearing aids were dead, weak, scratchy, intermittent, or squealing.

6.   Family/Friend Involvement. Two experiences on what it is like to have a mild hearing impairment are provided. One includes listening to a tape of ten spoken words filtered to simulate mild hearing impairment; the participants write down the words they have heard. The other is filling in the blanks of a paragraph, as if parts were not heard.

7.   Listening Strategies. Communication strategies such as combining visual, auditory, and contextual cues are discussed. Additionally, suggestions are offered to the participants to assume a more assertive approach for informing others of their hearing loss and requesting others to accommodate them with minor adjustments in their listening environment to facilitate the communicative process.

8.   Support Services. Describe local and national services available to hearing impaired persons. Organizations include Self Help for Hard of Hearing (SHHH), Voice, Minnesota Foundation for Better Hearing and Speech, and Regional Service Centers.

9.   Handouts. Direct the participant to the handouts which contain general information, and information on the support services.

Report Format:
The audiologist managing the patient should indicate in a chart note that the patient has attended the orientation session.

Billing:
No charge if the hearing aids are purchased through the University Affiliated Audiology Program.
If the hearing aids are obtained through Medical Assistance or purchased elsewhere, bill 2 units of Hearing Rehabilitation (CPT 92507).

References:
Davis, J. M., & Hardick, E. J. (1981). *Rehabilitative Audiology for Children and Adults.* New York: John Wiley & Sons.

Giolas, T. G. (1994). Aural rehabilitation of adults with hearing impairment. In J. Katz (Ed.) *Handbook of Clinical Audiology* (pp. 776-792). Baltimore, MD: Williams & Wilkins.

Hodgson, W. R. (1994). Audiologic Counseling. In J. Katz (Ed.) *Handbook of Clinical Audiology* (pp. 616-623). Baltimore, MD: Williams & Wilkins.

Skinner, M. W. (1988). *Hearing Aid Evaluation.* Englewood Cliffs, NJ: Prentice Hall.

Montano, J. (1994).   Rehabilitation technology for the hearing impaired.   In J. Katz (Ed.) *Handbook of Clinical Audiology* (pp. 638-654). Baltimore, MD: Williams & Wilkins.

National Association for Hearing and Speech Action, 10801 Rockville Pike, Rockville, Maryland 20852 (Religious places with amplifiers).

Nabelek, A. K., & Nabelek, I. V. (1994). Room acoustics and speech perception. In J. Katz (Ed.) *Handbook of Clinical Audiology* (pp. 624-637). Baltimore, MD: Williams & Wilkins.

Protocol 11 Annual (Hearing Aid) Review

Target Population:
Patients fit with hearing aids one or more years prior to the Annual Review visit.

Rationale:
The Annual Review is the final step in the one-year, hearing-aid delivery program. Subsequent reviews are performed at the patient's request or audiologist's suggestion. The goals of the Annual Review are:

    1. to determine whether the patient's hearing has changed significantly since previous testing;

    2. to determine whether the hearing aid continues to function appropriately and optimally; and

    3. to determine whether the patient is using the hearing aid to maximum advantage.

Equipment Required:
Electroacoustic hearing-aid analyzer with real-ear capabilities
Clinical audiometer with calibrated soundfield
Programmable hearing instrument equipment
Listening tube or stethoset
Grinding and buffing tools
Wax loop and brush
Magnifying glass
Battery tester
Screwdriver
Telephone
Otoscope

Methods:
Prior to the visit, a reminder letter will be sent to the patient. The hearing aid will be evaluated following the Annual Review Checklist (see Appendix):

1. <u>Patient's Interim History</u>. The audiologist will inquire as to whether the patient has noted significant changes in hearing, tinnitus, or dizziness and whether the patient has experienced any ear-related diseases or injuries, or changes in medications over the past year.

2. <u>Patient's Subjective Evaluation</u>. The audiologist should explore the quality of the patient's experience with the hearing aid. Among the considerations should be: whether the hearing aid is functioning adequately with respect to general function, loudness, sound quality, word recognition, and telephone usage. Inquiries should be directed towards discovering problems with feedback, moisture, intermittency, and difficult listening situations.

3.   Testing.
   a.   Air-Conduction Audiometry.   The audiologist will obtain a pure-tone, air-conduction audiogram.   If air-conduction thresholds have changed (or if the patient thinks his word-recognition abilities have changed), a complete hearing evaluation should be considered.   The patient should be informed that fees for testing beyond the air-conduction audiogram are not covered by the dispensing fee.
   b.   Electroacoustic Check.   The hearing aid should be checked electroacoustically at use and/or full-on gain settings.   Refer to Protocol 12 Electroacoustic Hearing Aid Evaluation.
   c.   Real-ear Gain or Functional Gain.   Real-Ear Insertion Response (REIR) or functional gain should be measured if the patient's hearing has changed, if significant physical modifications are made in the hearing aid, if acoustic parameters are changed, or if the volume control is set to greater than one-half on. Refer to Protocol 8 Hearing Aid Fitting (Methods, #2).

4.   Audiologist's Observations. The audiologist will check the physical fit of the hearing aid or earmold, the sound bore and vents for wax, and earmold and tubing for shrinkage, yellowing, stiffness, or cracks.   The patient's ears should also be inspected for cerumen.   The audiologist will listen to the hearing aid checking for sound quality, feedback, internal noise, and intermittency with and without pressure applied to the case and/or battery compartment.   The trimmers and volume control should be rotated listening for dead spots.   Additionally, the battery contacts should be checked for integrity and corrosion.   The audiologist will evaluate hearing aid settings for appropriate use and reserve gain.

5.   Battery Life. The record of battery life should be consistent with use schedule and expected battery drain.

6.   Modifications.   A careful record should be kept of any changes.
   a.   Hearing Aid Settings. The audiologist will document the initial settings for each aid and any changes made at the time of the Annual Review.
   b.   Physical Modification.   A physical adjustment of the instrument may be necessary.   This may include grinding and buffing for a more comfortable fit in the ear, vent enlargement for modification of frequency response or control of occlusion effect.

7.   Recommendations.   Recommendations for medical follow-up and/or audiological evaluations should be discussed with the patient.   If the hearing aid is not functioning adequately, the audiologist should determine whether a response modification, new instrument, repair, or second aid may be beneficial.

8.   Return Appointment. Recommendations for return appointments should be recorded on the checklist. Reminder postcards will be self-addressed by those patients requiring annual or semi-annual follow-up appointments.

Report Format:
Audiogram (including any functional gain results) - original in hospital and copy in dispensing chart.
Annual Review Checklist - original in dispensing chart.
Real-ear measurement results - original in dispensing chart.
Chart Note - in hospital chart if significant hearing change occurred or if significant problems

exist, and in dispensary chart. Indicate reason for appointment in both hospital and dispensary charts.

Billing:
There is no charge for a first year annual review. Any additional hearing testing beyond an air-conduction audiogram should be billed appropriately. There is no charge for repair through 1 year beyond invoice/ship date if the hearing aid is fit through this clinic. Bill for any services provided beyond the first year.

References:
Skinner, M. W. (1988). *Hearing Aid Evaluation.* Englewood Cliffs, NJ: Prentice Hall.

Protocol 11 Appendix

Annual Review Checklist

ANNUAL REVIEW CHECKLIST

Examiner	Date	Birthdate

	Manufacturer	Model	Serial Number
R			
L			
Rem			
Ctrl			

Patient's Interim History

		Worse	Same	Better	NA
Hearing	R	☐	☐	☐	☐
	L	☐	☐	☐	☐
Tinnitus	R	☐	☐	☐	☐
	L	☐	☐	☐	☐
Vertigo		☐	☐	☐	☐

☐ Diseases _____
☐ Injury _____
☐ Medication _____

Patient's Subjective Evaluation

		Adequate	Inadequate
General Function	R	☐	☐
	L	☐	☐
Loudness	R	☐	☐
	L	☐	☐
Sound Quality	R	☐	☐
	L	☐	☐
Word Recognition	R	☐	☐
	L	☐	☐

☐ Telephone _____
☐ Feedback _____
☐ Moisture / Intermittency _____
☐ Wax _____
☐ Other _____

Use Schedule / Battery Life

	Curr Dr (mA)	Exp Hrs/day	Act Hrs/day
R			
L			

Testing

☐ Air Cond Thresholds _____
☐ Electroacoustics_____
☐ Functional Gain _____
☐ Real Ear Gain_____

Audiologist's Observations

☐ Physical Fit _____
☐ Wax _____
☐ Clarity/Quality _____
☐ Feedback _____
☐ Internal Noise _____
☐ Volume Setting _____
☐ Battery Drawer _____
☐ Earmold Integrity _____
☐ Other _____

Conventional Settings

Initial ◯ ◯ ◯ ◯ ◯ ◯
_____ _____ _____ _____ _____ _____

Final ◯ ◯ ◯ ◯ ◯ ◯
_____ _____ _____ _____ _____ _____

Programmable Settings

Initial _____
_____

Final _____
_____

Physical Modifications

☐ Shell _____
☐ Earmold _____
☐ Other _____

Recommendations

☐ Medical Review_____
☐ Hearing Aid_____
☐ Postcard Apptmt Reminder _____
☐ Other _____
_____
_____
_____

Protocol 12 Electroacoustic Hearing Aid Evaluation

Target Population:
Electroacoustic Hearing-Aid Evaluations can be performed in conjunction with initial fitting, fitting follow-ups, annual reviews, refits after repair, ENT consultations (time permitting and pending patient's permission), and patient visits where the initial fitting or repair took place outside the clinic. All hearing aids destined for patient use as loaners or demonstrators are candidates for an Electroacoustic Hearing-Aid Evaluation. An Electroacoustic Hearing-Aid Evaluation should be performed on any instrument when there are questions about its performance.

Rationale:
The objective of making electroacoustic measurements on hearing aids is to provide data that are useful in selecting or adjusting a hearing aid for a particular impaired ear. These data are used to:

    a.   evaluate compliance with the manufacturer's specifications,

    b.   verify the degree of success in meeting prescriptive frequency-response characteristics.

Equipment Required:
Hearing aid batteries or a battery substitute
Hearing aid battery tester or voltmeter
Hearing aid listening tube
Hearing aid analyzer (Fonix 6500, Virtual M340 or equivalent)

Methods:
The choice of test protocol depends on the specific objective. Step 1 should be performed in all cases before proceeding. Step 2a should be performed on all new or repaired hearing aids to determine if the aid performs within manufacturer and ANSI specifications. Step 2b is performed at the discretion of the audiologist to evaluate the extent to which the hearing aid is appropriate for the patient. Refer to the protocol on hearing-aid fittings (Protocol 8) for specific test objectives for step 2b.

1.   Clean the surface of all hearing aids with an alcohol wipe before proceeding with any listening or electroacoustic check. Ensure that a fresh battery is in the hearing aid. Listen to the aid to determine if it works and if the gain (i.e. volume) control varies the output level. Listen for gross distortion, intermittency, and noise. Check for cerumen in the receiver ports of custom instruments.

2.   ANSI standard electroacoustic evaluation.

a.   Obtain data pursuant to ANSI S3.22 1987. All vents should be plugged at both ends for this testing. All trimmers should be set to provide the widest frequency response and the greatest gain and output possible. Automatic-gain control (AGC) aids should be set for linear operation and tested as a linear aid (if a control is available), or set for maximum AGC action and tested as an AGC aid (if only a kneepoint trimmer is available). Tests to be performed are as follows:

Test Description ANSI S3.22	Section	ANSI Terminology
Saturation Sound Press. Level Curve (SSPL90)	6.2	FREQ SWEEP
Full-On Gain Curve (FOG)	3.7, 3.8, 6.4, 6.5	FREQ SWEEP
Max. Saturation Sound Press. Level	6.2	MAX SSPL
High-Frequency Average -SSPL90	3.5, 3.6, 6.3	HF AVG SSPL
HFA Full-On Gain	3.7, 3.8, 6.4, 6.5	HF AVG GAIN
Reference-Test Gain	3.9, 3.10, 6.6, 6.7	REF TEST GAIN
Total-Harmonic Distortion	6.11	THD, ALT FREQ
Equivalent-Input Noise Level (L_n)	6.12	INPUT NOISE
Battery Current	6.13	CURRENT DRAIN

b.   Obtain response data using ANSI measurement protocols as above, with the gain control and trimmers set either in the patient's use positions, or at experimental settings as desired by the audiologist. Tests are chosen at the audiologist's discretion. Examples include: multiple SSPL90, FOG, and frequency-response curves with appropriate trimmers at extremes of adjustment, telecoil, AGC, attack/release times, total-harmonic distortion tests, etc.

Report Format:
Hearing-aid electroacoustic measurement results are placed in the dispensing chart.
Examples of printouts for the Fonix 6500 and Virtual M340 are included as Appendices A and B, respectively.

Billing:
No charge when performed during the first year for hearing aids purchased through the clinic, except for insurance plans which pay for visits separately.
Otherwise: Bill one Electroacoustic Hearing-Aid Test unit per aid tested. When the primary purpose of the appointment is to recheck hearing, bill accordingly for the audiologic evaluation and charge Hearing Rehabilitation (CPT 92507) or Hearing Consultation (CPT 99242) unit(s) for the time spent performing electroacoustic tests.

References:
 American National Standards Institute. (1987). *American National Standard Specification for Hearing Aid Measurements.* (ANSI S3.22-1987). New York.

American National Standards Institute. (1992). *Testing Hearing Aids with a Broad Band Noise Signal.* (ANSI S3.42-1992). New York.

Lybarger, S. F. (1985). The physical and electroacoustic characteristics of hearing aids. In J. Katz (Ed.), *Handbook of Clinical Audiology* (pp. 849-884). Baltimore, MD: Williams and Wilkins.

Protocol 12 Appendix

A.   Fonix Electroacoustic Printout
B.   Virtual M340 Electroacoustic Printout

FONIX ELECTROACOUSTIC PRINTOUT

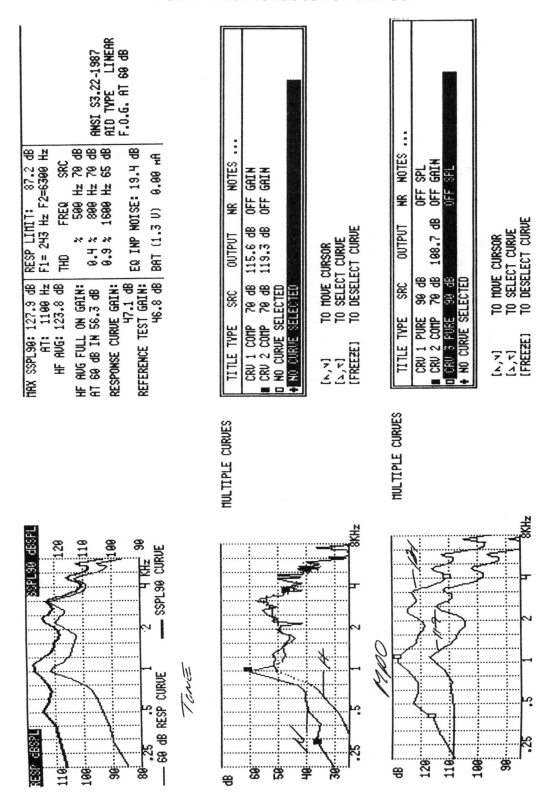

MAX SSPL90: 127.9 dB
AT: 1100 Hz
HF AVG: 123.8 dB

RESP LIMIT: 87.2 dB
F1= 243 Hz F2=6300 Hz

THD   FREQ   SRC
      %   500 Hz 70 dB
 0.4 %   800 Hz 70 dB
 0.9 % 1600 Hz 65 dB

HF AVG FULL ON GAIN:
AT 60 dB IN 56.3 dB
RESPONSE CURVE GAIN:
              47.1 dB
REFERENCE TEST GAIN:
              46.8 dB

EQ INP NOISE: 19.4 dB
BAT (1.3 V) 0.00 mA

ANSI S3.22-1987
AID TYPE   LINEAR
F.O.G. AT 60 dB

MULTIPLE CURVES

TITLE	TYPE	SRC	OUTPUT	NR	NOTES ...
CRV 1 COMP	70 dB	115.6 dB	OFF GAIN
CRV 2 COMP	70 dB	119.3 dB	OFF GAIN
NO CURVE SELECTED
NO CURVE SELECTED

[∧,∨]   TO MOVE CURSOR
[∆,∇]   TO SELECT CURVE
[FREEZE] TO DESELECT CURVE

MULTIPLE CURVES

TITLE	TYPE	SRC	OUTPUT	NR	NOTES ...
CRV 1 PURE	90 dB	OFF SPL
CRV 2 COMP	70 dB	108.7 dB	OFF GAIN
CRV 3 PURE	90 dB	OFF SPL
NO CURVE SELECTED

[∧,∨]   TO MOVE CURSOR
[∆,∇]   TO SELECT CURVE
[FREEZE] TO DESELECT CURVE

VIRTUAL M340 ELECTROACOUSTIC PRINTOUT

UMHC Audiology Clinic, Univ. of Minn.
Box 283 UMHC-516 Delaware St. SE
Minneapolis, MN 55455 Suite 8-106
(612) 626-5775

Patient: Stock Aid
Audiologist:
Number:
Sex: Male Age:
Saturday, August 10, 1996
Virtual Model 340 Probe-Microphone System

Right Aid Type: Left Aid Type:
Right Aid Settings: Left Aid Settings:
Right Aid Number: Left Aid Number:
Right Earmold: Left Earmold:

Right Ear ANSI test results

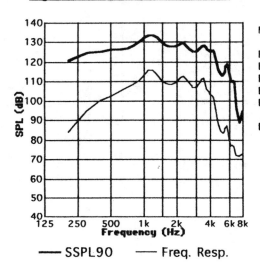

Max SSPL90:	131.8	dB
At:	1100	Hz
HF Average-SSPL90:	127.6	dB
HF Average-Full Gain:	62.7	dB
Reference Test Gain:	50.6	dB
Equiv. Noise, L_n:	21.0	dB
Response Limit:	89.6	dB
f1 = 300 Hz, f2 =	4800	Hz
Battery Current:	0.0	mA

Freq (Hz)	THD (%)	Source:
500	1.7	70 dB
800	0.6	70 dB
1600	0.5	65 dB

———— SSPL90   ——— Freq. Resp.

Right Ear Sound Chamber Test

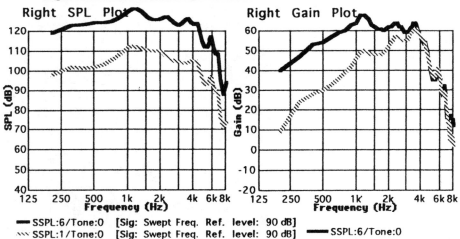

■—SSPL:6/Tone:0   [Sig: Swept Freq. Ref. level: 90 dB]
ⁿⁿⁿ SSPL:1/Tone:0   [Sig: Swept Freq. Ref. level: 90 dB]

■—SSPL:6/Tone:0
ⁿⁿⁿ SSPL:6/Tone:5

Section III
Physiological Assessment of Auditory System

Protocol 13 ABR Neurologic Evaluation

Target Population:
Patients whose symptomatology or audiological results suggest the possibility of retrocochlear pathology. Things to consider are unexplained asymmetrical sensorineural hearing loss, unilateral tinnitus, dizziness, unexplained feeling of fullness in the ear, poor word recognition scores, word recognition rollover, acoustic reflex thresholds inconsistent with pure tone results, or positive acoustic reflex decay.

Rationale:
Lesions of the auditory pathway may increase the latency and decrease the amplitudes of the auditory brainstem response (ABR) waves. Since these lesions are almost always unilateral, a comparison of ABR results with those from the contralateral ear provides information that is useful in the diagnosis of retrocochlear lesions.

Equipment Required:
Otoscope
Surface electrodes (e.g., disposable adhesive electrodes with snap-on electrode leads)
Insert earphones with gold-foil wrapped canal electrodes
Evoked potential system
Materials for applying electrodes
       alcohol swabs, skin preparatory materials, e.g. Nu-prep™ or OMNI-PREP®, gauze pads,
       conductive gel or cream
Comfortable reclining chair or cot

Methods:
1.   The electrode configuration is: active: forehead or vertex
                                        reference: ipsilateral ear canal
                                          ground: contralateral ear canal
Ear canal electrodes are preferred because they provide superior recordings of Wave I. If ear canal electrodes cannot be used, earlobe or mastoid electrodes may be used.

2.   Otoscopic inspection. The ear canals should be clear so that the canal electrodes can make good contact with the ear canal epithelium and the sound bore does not become occluded. If there is excessive cerumen, the ear canals should be cleaned. (See Protocol 3 Cerumen Removal.)

3.   Apply a surface electrode to the vertex or high forehead area.
     a.   Clean skin with alcohol pad.
     b.   Using a gauze pad moistened with preparatory gel, rub skin until it is pink.

c.   Apply electrode insuring that it adheres well to the skin. If it does not, it can be secured with tape.

d.   Use disk electrodes if the condition of the skin precludes the use of adhesive electrodes or if adhesive electrodes do not securely adhere to the skin.

4.   Insert the canal electrodes, moistened with electrode cream, into the ear canals until nearly all the plug is within the canal. Apply slight pressure and hold for 20 seconds while the foam plug expands.

5.   Plug the electrodes into the patient connection box and measure electrode impedances. Record impedances on the ABR/ECOG Worksheet (Appendix A).

6.   Select appropriate stimulus and data collection parameters (Appendix B).

7.   Stimulating the better ear, simultaneously record the ABR for 80 dBnHL rarefaction and condensation clicks, accumulating separate averages for the two polarities (1500 repetitions for each polarity, 38 clicks/s). These can be added to obtain the alternating polarity response. Collect at least 2 averages which show replicable waves I, III, & V. Reverse the ear canal electrode connections so that the poorer ear can be tested. Again collect at least two averages which show replicable waves I, III, & V. Use contralateral masking when appropriate. For each recording, enter stimulus and recording conditions on ABR/ECOG Worksheet.

8.   The following suggestions may help you to obtain good quality averages.
a.   For noisy records, talk to the patient to find out how to make him/her more comfortable and encourage him/her to relax.
b.   If the signal-to-noise ratio is poor, average more sweeps.
c.   If a large proportion of responses are rejected by the artifact rejection system, it may be necessary to reduce the amplifier gain or raise the artifact reject threshold.
d.   To enhance wave I, slow the repetition rate to 13/sec. If wave I is still not obtained a tympanic membrane electrode can be used (Protocol 16)
e.   To enhance all waves, increase intensity of stimulus. When changing click intensity, the masker level may need to be changed also.

9.   Interpretation. Interaural interpeak (I-III or I-V) latency differences exceeding 0.30 ms or absent wave III and/or V should be interpreted as evidence of retrocochlear pathology. If latencies from the non-test ear cannot be obtained use one of the following as an indicator of retrocochlear pathology: I-V interpeak latency > 4.3 ms; wave V latency > 6.3 ms (0.8 ms sound tube delay subtracted).

Report Format:
Patient identification, waveforms, latencies and interwave latencies should be printed out on the Auditory Evoked Potentials Form (see Appendix C). Waveforms should be labeled as to ear stimulated, click intensity, repetition rate, and click polarity used. Any changes from standard protocol must also be recorded on the form and any other information that may be useful in interpretation may be added. The results should be summarized in a chart note or a statement such as "no evidence of retrocochlear pathology" or "retrocochlear pathology can not be ruled out" should be written on the form.

Billing:
Bill Auditory Brainstem Response Audiometry (CPT 92585 or CPT 92599 if sedated) in 15 minute units and Clinic Visit in 15 minute units.

References:
ASHA, Audiologic Evaluation Working Group on Auditory Evoked Potential Measurements. (1987). *The Short Latency Auditory Evoked Potentials* (pp. 1-8; 16-26). Rockville, MD: ASHA.

Durrant, J. D., & Wolf, K. E. (1991). Auditory evoked potentials: Basic aspects. In W. F. Rintelmann (Ed.), *Hearing Assessment* (pp. 321-382). Austin, TX: Pro-Ed.

Hall, J. W. III. (1992). *Handbook of Auditory Evoked Potentials*. Boston: Allyn and Bacon.

Jacobson, J. T. (Ed.) (1985). *The Auditory Brainstem Response*. San Diego: College-Hill Press.

Musiek, F. E. (1991). Auditory evoked responses in site of lesion assessment. In W. F. Rintelmann (Ed.), *Hearing Assessment* (pp. 383-428). Austin, TX: Pro-Ed.

Musiek, F. E., Bornstein, S. P., Hall, J. W., & Schwaber, M. K. (1994). Auditory brainstem response: neurodiagnostic and intraoperative applications. In J. Katz (Ed.), *Handbook of Clinical Audiology* (pp. 351-374). Baltimore: Williams & Wilkins.

Protocol 13 Appendix

AUDITORY BRAINSTEM RESPONSE / ELECTROCOCHLEOGRAPHY WORKSHEET

NAME: _____   HOSP. ID _____

BIRTHDATE   ___-___-___   DATE   ___-___-___

		R		L	
	CH1	CH2	CH1	CH2	CH1	CH2
ELECTRODE MONTAGE: ACTIVE ___ ___	ELECTRODE IMPEDANCE ___	___	___	___
REFERENCE ___ ___	___	___	___	___
GROUND ___ ___	___	___	___	___

RECORD	EAR	TRANS-DUCER	STIM	RISE	DUR	POLARITY	RATE	LEVEL	# SWEEPS	GAIN	WINDOW	FILTERS
1												
2												
3												
4												
5												
6												
7												
8												
9												
10												
11												
12												
13												
14												
15												
16												
17												
18												
19												
20												
21												

SET-UP FOR AUDITORY BRAINSTEM RESPONSE THRESHOLDS

Connecting electrodes:
The active electrode should be plugged into CH 1 - ACT, the reference electrode into CH 1 - REF, and the ground electrode into GND on the electrode connection box.

Parameter setup:
1.   Ear stimulated (right or left); electrode connections will also have to change.
2   Intensity level in dB nHL; normally 90 dB is the starting level, however if the threshold at 2000 Hz is 50 dB or worse, increase to 88 dB (the maximum level). When the click level is raised to 90 dB, raise the masker level from 30 dB to 40 dB. When changing click level, be sure to change level for both polarities.
3.   Rate may be changed from 38/s to 13/s or 70/s.
4   Amplifier gain may be changed from 100,000 to 75,000 or 50,000 to allow response collection in the presence of large artifacts. (See Step 8c.)

Parameter Setup Screen

GENERAL SETUP
Test: P300
Channels: 1
Window: 10.000
Pre/Post: 0
Points: 256

AMPLIFIER SETUP
Gain: 100000
Hi Filter: 1500
Low Filter: 100.00
Notch filter: out
Artifact: enabled
Electrodes: Fz/Ec/Ec

STIMULUS SETUP
Stimulator: Insert   Type: condensing click   80 dB
Max # Stim.: 1500
Rate (/s): 38.0   Ear: left   mask: white   30 dB
P300 ratio: 1
infrequent stim: rarefacting click   80 dB

AUDITORY EVOKED POTENTIALS FORM

UNIVERSITY OF MINNESOTA HOSPITAL AND CLINIC
AUDIOLOGY CLINIC
AUDITORY EVOKED POTENTIALS

EXAMINER *J Hirsch*   DATE *7-17-96*   PATIENT BIRTHDATE *12-18-59*

☑ AUDITORY BRAINSTEM RESPONSE (ABR)
☐ TYMPANIC ELECTROCOCHLEOGRAPHY
☐ TRANSTYMPANIC ELECTROCOCHLEOGRAPHY
☐ INTRAOPERATIVE MONITORING

Hospital ID#
Patient Name

Patient:
Address:
            Austin,   MN
Phone   : Neurol.

Born: 12/18/59   Age: 0 year(s)
File: SL102794   ID #:
Physician:
Operator : JH   Date: 07/17/96

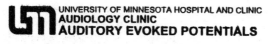

Left ear   *Clicks*   *Right ear*
                  38/s
        I   III   V   I   III   V   *rarefaction*
A1 .25uV   *rarefaction*   *80dBnHL*   A7 .25uV
A2 .25uV   *80dBnHL*   *80dB*   A8 .25uV
                  80dB

        I   III   V   III
A3 .25uV   *Condensation*   I   *Condensation*   A5 .25uV
A4 .25uV   *80dBnHL*   V *80dBnHL*   A6 .25uV
                  80dB   *80dB*

LATENCY   2.00 ms/div

LATENCY OFFSET   -.80 ms

LATENCIES (ms)

	I	II	III	IV	V	VI	VII	VIII	IX	X
B1	1.54		3.89		5.65	*Left*
B3	1.70		3.93		5.65	"
B5	1.78		3.85		5.65	*Right*
B7	1.62		3.85		5.41	"

No evidence of
retrocochlear pathology.

Protocol 14 ABR Threshold Evaluation

Target Population:
Patients who cannot be tested by behavioral audiometry or whose results are incomplete or ambiguous following behavioral testing. Patients who fail infant hearing screening (Protocol 15) are tested for ABR thresholds. ABR threshold evaluation is also useful for intraoperative assessment of hearing sensitivity, such as during middle ear reconstructive surgery.

Rationale:
ABR results are used to assess hearing sensitivity in the 500, 1000, 2000, and 4000-Hz frequency regions for each ear. Bone conduction thresholds may also be determined in cases where a conductive loss is suspected.

Equipment Required:
Otoscope
Evoked potential system
Otoacoustic emission system
Surface electrodes (disposable adhesive electrodes with snap-on leads)
Insert earphones or headphones
Bone vibrator
Materials for applying electrodes
Alcohol swabs, skin preparatory materials e.g., NuPrep™ or OMNI-PREP®, gauze pads, conductive gel or cream
Comfortable reclining chair, cot, or crib
Blanket, pillow, pacifier, juice, nipple, and spare diapers
Pediatric ambu (resuscitation bag)
Stethoscope

Methods:
1.   Otoscopic inspection. The ear canals should be clear so that the sound is not attenuated. A small amount of wax may also occlude the bore of the insert phone. If there is excessive cerumen, the ear canals should be cleaned. (See Protocol 3 Cerumen Removal.)

2.   Assess cochlear function by obtaining click-evoked otoacoustic emissions (80 dB SPL clicks) or distortion product emissions (70 dB SPL f1 & f2 tones) in the 1500-6000 Hz range (see TEOAE Screen Protocol 15). If emissions are clearly present in both ears you may choose not to continue with the ABR testing or you may limit the testing to an ABR threshold screening, using rarefaction clicks presented at 70 and 30 dB nHL, and/or obtaining 500-Hz tone burst thresholds.

3.   Determine ABR thresholds.
        a.   If sedation is required see information in Appendix A.

b.   Electrode configuration: active: forehead or vertex
                                          reference: ipsilateral mastoid
                                          ground: contralateral mastoid

Apply electrodes as follows:
          1.   clean skin with alcohol pad
          2.   using a gauze pad moistened with abrasive solution, rub skin until it is
pink
          3.   apply self-adhesive electrode; if electrode does not adhere well to the
skin, it can be secured with tape. Conductive gel or cream may be added to
moisten electrode.
c.   Plug the electrodes into the patient connection box and record impedances on the
ABR/ECOG Worksheet (Appendix B).
d.   Set up acquisition parameters and record on ABR/ECOG Worksheet, maintaining a
record of each trial. See Appendix C and D for specific setup parameters for each type of
stimulus. See Appendix E for threshold evaluation flow chart.
e.   Using rarefaction click stimulation, collect one response at 70 dB nHL and if the
waves are easily identifiable, collect 1-2 responses at 30 dB nHL. If no response is seen
at 70 dB, increase the intensity to 80 dB nHL and then to 90 dB nHL. If no response is
seen at 80 or 90 dB nHL, or the stimulus artifact interferes too much to see a response,
try using alternating polarity clicks and/or a slower rate. If the threshold is 85 dB or
greater, skip to step 9. If a response was present at 70 dB or less obtain thresholds for
1000, 2000, and 4000-Hz tone bursts.
f.   Using alternating 4000-Hz tone bursts obtain a response at 70 dB nHL. If no
response is seen, increase the intensity to 80 and then 100 dB nHL to obtain a threshold.
If a response is present at 70 dB, decrease the level to 30 dB and continue to decrease the
level in 10 dB steps until no response is seen. If no response was seen at 30 dB, obtain a
response at 50 dB; then test either at 60 or 40 dB nHL depending on whether a response
was present at 50 dB. It is advisable to replicate responses whenever the recordings are
noisy or there is any doubt about the presence of a response.
g.   Follow the same procedure using 1000 and/or 2000-Hz tone bursts starting at
70 dB nHL.
h.   Using a rarefaction 500-Hz tone burst (2 ms rise-fall, 2 ms plateau), collect a
response at 50 dB nHL and if the response is identifiable, collect responses, decreasing
the intensity in 10 dB steps, until no response is seen. If no response is seen at 50 dB
nHL, increase the intensity in 20 dB steps until a response is seen.
i.   Reverse reference and ground electrode leads. Repeat steps 6-9 for the opposite
ear. Begin with the 30 dB nHL stimulus if there is concern of the patient waking up. If
the responses are very clear at lower levels there may be no need to test at the louder
levels.
j.   Obtain tympanograms for each ear as described in Protocol 1, Basic Hearing
Evaluation.
k.   If the tympanograms are not normal and/or all waves are delayed in responses to
clicks $\geq$ 50 dB nHL, bone-conducted thresholds should be obtained. Because of the
limited range of intensities possible, begin at the highest level and decrease in 20-dB
steps until no response is seen. Collect another response 10 dB higher than the level at
which there is no response. If the stimulus artifact interferes too much to see a
response, the bone vibrator may be placed on the mastoid to which the ground electrode
is connected. Masking should be provided if ear specific information is needed.
l.   Use the following guidelines to estimate audiometric thresholds:

1.   For clicks and 1000, 2000 and 4000-Hz tone bursts, threshold is estimated at 5 dB below the lowest level at which a response is seen.

2.   For 500-Hz tone bursts, the audiometric threshold is estimated at 15 dB below the lowest level at which a response is seen. If the patient is in a deep sleep, Wave V may be identifiable at supra-threshold intensity levels. At near-threshold levels, however, the identifiable response may appear as a shallow negative trough at a latency slightly larger than that of Wave V at higher levels. Threshold estimated at 15 dB better than the lowest level at which the negative trough can be identified.

3.   For bone-conducted clicks, thresholds are no worse than the lowest level at which a response is seen. A 0.5 msec. delay in the bone-conducted wave V latencies, compared to air-conducted wave V latencies for the same stimulus, has been reported. This delay has not been explained, but may be due to transducer phase differences. Otherwise the latency-intensity curves are similar to those for air conduction clicks.

4.   For bone-conducted 500-Hz tone bursts, use the guidelines in 13b.

5.   Comparing the latencies of wave V to age-specific latency-intensity norms (Gorga, et al., 1989) may help determine whether the loss is conductive or sensorineural. The normal ranges are based on responses from rarefaction clicks. However, response latencies to the 2000 or 4000-Hz tone bursts can be plotted if the rise time of the stimulus is subtracted from the wave V latency.

m.   The following suggestions may help you to obtain good quality averages.

1.   For noisy records, try to make the patient more comfortable.

2.   Average more sweeps.

3.   If a high proportion of responses are being rejected by the artifact reject system, it maybe necessary to reduce the amplifier gain or raise the artifact reject threshold.

4.   If there is any doubt about the presence of a response, do a silent control (-5 dB HL) to determine the noise level.

Report Format:
Patient identification, waveforms, and latencies should be printed on the Auditory Evoked Potentials Form (see Appendix F). Waveforms should be labeled as to ear stimulated, type of stimulus, intensity, and repetition rate. Any changes from standard protocol must also be recorded and any other information that may be useful in interpretation may be added. The wave V latency-intensity function should be plotted on the appropriate latency-intensity confidence limit graph and attached to the waveform printout (see Appendix G and Protocol 15, Appendix D). Fill out the ABR Threshold Evaluation Form (see Appendix H) which summarizes all the evaluation information.
A written report should be sent to referring sources.

Billing:
Bill for Auditory Brainstem Response Audiometry (CPT 92585 or CPT 92599 if sedated) in 15-minute units.

References:
ASHA, Audiologic Evaluation Working Group on Auditory Evoked Potential Measurements. (1987). *The Short Latency Auditory Evoked Potentials* (pp. 1-8; 16-26). Rockville, MD: ASHA.

Gorga, M., & Thornton, A. (1989). The choice of stimuli for ABR measurements. *Ear and Hearing, 10,* 217-230.

Gorga, M., Worthington, D., Reiland, J., Beauchaine, K., & Goldgar, D. (1985). Some comparisons between auditory brainstem response thresholds, latencies and the pure-tone audiogram. *Ear and Hearing, 6,* 105-112.

Gorga, M., Kaminski, J., Beauchaine, K., Jesteadt, W., & Neely, S. (1989). Auditory brainstem responses from children three months to three years of age: Normal patterns of response II. *Journal of Speech and Hearing Research, 32,* 281-288.

Hall, J. W. III. (1992). *Handbook of Auditory Evoked Potentials.* Boston: Allyn & Bacon.

Keith, W., & Greville, A. (1987) Effects of Audiometric Configuration on the Auditory Brain Stem Response. *Ear and Hearing, 8,* 49-55.

Liston, S. L., Levine, S. C., Margolis, R., H., & Yanz, J. L. (1991). Use of intraoperative ABR to guide prosthesis positioning. *Laryngoscope, 101,* 1009-1012.

Schwartz, D. M., & Schwartz, J. A. (1991). Auditory evoked potentials in clinical pediatrics. In W. F. Rintelmann (Ed.), *Hearing Assessment* (pp. 429-476). Austin, TX: Pro-Ed.

Weber, B. A. (1994). Auditory brainstem response: Threshold evaluation and auditory screening. In J. Katz (Ed.), *Handbook of Clinical Audiology*, 4th ed. (pp. 375-386). Baltimore: Williams & Wilkins.

Protocol 14 Appendix

A.   Sedation Information
B.   Auditory Brainstem Response/Electrocochleography Worksheet
C.   Parameters for Click Thresholds
D.   Parameters for Toneburst Thresholds
E.   Threshold Evaluation Flowchart
F.   Auditory Brainstem Response Audiometry Form
G.   Latency/Intensity Function Example
H.   Auditory Brainstem Response Threshold Evaluation

GUIDELINES FOR SEDATION FOR AUDITORY BRAINSTEM RESPONSE TESTING

Infants under 4 months of age rarely need sedation as the ABR thresholds can be obtained while the infant sleeps. Children from 4 months to 4 years of age can be sedated with chloral hydrate. for children for whom chloral hydrate has been ineffective and for children older than 4, stronger sedation e.g. seconal or a combination of Demerol, Thorazine, and Phenergan may be necessary.

Procedure for chloral hydrate.

1.   Obtain a written sedation order and schedule a nurse for monitoring the child. (See Standard Orders for Pediatric Sedation.)

2.   Send ABR information and feeding and sleeping instructions to the parents. (See Auditory Brainstem Response (ABR) Audiometry - Some Common Questions and Answers.)

3.   The nurse's responsibilities are to:
        a.   weigh the child and administer the sedation,
        b.   monitor pulse and respiration rate and child's color, recording the information every 15 minutes,
        c.   wake the child and see that the child can take fluids,
        d.   give verbal discharge instructions to the parents, as well as written instructions. (See Discharge Instructions Following Sedation.)

Procedure for other sedations.

Child will be admitted to the Day Hospital or other short stay unit for care and monitoring.

PHYSICIAN'S ORDERS (STANDING ORDERS)

ORIGINATED BY (PHYSICIAN)	ORIGINATED	REVISED

TITLE: **STANDARD ORDERS FOR PEDIATRIC SEDATION**   wt: 10 kg

Specific Allergies: _Neda_

Procedures: _ABR_

Procedure Date: _7-19-96_

Check appropriate orders:

_4_   Chloral Hydrate 50-80 mg/kg PO 30 minutes before procedure.

_4_   May repeat above x 1 prn.

    Demerol 1 mg/kg +

    Thorazine 0.5 mg/kg +

    Phenergan 0.5 mg/kg + IM 30 minutes before procedure

    Other (attach script):

    Start peripheral IV with Normal Saline TKO.

    Monitor patient post procedure.

_4_   May discharge to home when awake and able to tolerate fluids.

Physician Signature:

Nurse's Notes: 12^N Chloral hydrate 500 mg given po. p 122 R 26

    12^{20}p child sleeping soundly. P 118 R 26. ABR testing began

    12^{35} : P 118 R 24 12^{50}p P 110 R 24 Child continues to sleep. Color good.

    1^{05}p P 110 R 24 1^{20}p ABR testing completed

    Child awakened easily. PO'g apple juice. 2p D/c'd with post instructions

    to care of parents.

R.N Signature

AUDITORY BRAINSTEM RESPONSE (ABR) AUDIOMETRY
SOME COMMON QUESTIONS AND ANSWERS

1)   WHAT CAN WE EXPECT TO LEARN FROM ABR?

In the case of young children and others who are unable to tell us when they hear a sound, we can determine if the ear is receiving sound and sending it to the brain for interpretation. ABR will not tell us how the patient interprets sound once it reaches the brain.

2)   WHAT PREPARATION IS NEEDED FOR THE TEST?

In order to complete the testing, the child needs to remain very quiet and still. If the child is less than 2-4 months old, she/he will probably fall asleep while taking a bottle, and therefore the child should come to the clinic before feeding and nap time. for all other children, sedation is often used to help them sleep through the test. *The children should not be given anything to eat or drink within 3-4 hours of the test, and they should be deprived of their normal sleep.* That is, they should be deprived of any nap prior to the test, or for children scheduled for testing in the morning, they should be kept up later the night before the test and awakened earlier on the day of the test. *It is very important that the child, even an infant, does not sleep in the car on their way to the appointment.*

3)   ARE THERE ANY RISKS?

The sedation is administered by a nurse under medical supervision, after written authorization for sedation has been given by a doctor. Most children go to sleep with half an hour.

The test does not hurt. ABR is a safe procedure in which three electrodes are taped to the surface of the child's head, on the forehead and behind each ear. An earplug is placed in the ear canal for sounds to be presented to the ear. The child usually wake sleeps throughout the entire procedure, which averages around one hour. Parents are welcome to be present during the entire procedure.

If you have any questions, please feel free to contact the Audiology Clinic.

DISCHARGE INSTRUCTIONS FOLLOWING SEDATION

The sedative your child received today was _____ mg of _____ . A second dose of _____
was given at _____ for a total of _____ . In case your child should need sedation in
the future, keep this information with your health records. You will know what he or she has
received and how well it worked.

Some reminders:

It is normal for your child to be more sleepy and irritable today. Awaken your child every 1 to
1 1/2 hours today, if he/she continues to sleep. This is so your child will sleep throughout the
night.

If your child is a young infant, make sure the car seat or infant seat does not bend the child's
head forward and down so that it obstructs breathing.

Older children need to be supervised by an adult for activities which require balance. (Bike
riding, skate boarding, stair climbing should be avoided.)

When your child begins to eat again, start with liquids, such as juice, pop or popsicles. If your
child is not bothered by nausea, a regular diet may be resumed. However, light meals are
suggested. If nausea or vomiting occurs, give small amounts of clear liquids; for example, 7 Up,
apple juice or broth. Fluids are more important than food until your child is feeling better.

Some over-the-counter medications can contain alcohol, such as:
    Liquid cold/cough medications: Robitussin, Formula 44 for children.
    Liquid allergy medications: Benedryl, Chlortrimetron.
    Liquid pain medications: Tylenol, Panadol, Advil.

Please DO NOT GIVE THESE FOR AT LEAST 24 HOURS FOLLOWING CHLORAL HYDRATE.

If you plan to leave your child with a babysitter, your sitter should be given the same
instructions we have given you regarding your child's care.

If you have any questions or concerns, please call the following:
Audiology Clinic   Emergency Room

AUDITORY BRAINSTEM RESPONSE / ELECTROCOCHLEOGRAPHY WORKSHEET

NAME: _____   HOSP. ID _____

BIRTHDATE ____-____-____   DATE ____-____-____

		CH1	CH2				R CH1	CH2	L CH1	CH2
ELECTRODE MONTAGE:	ACTIVE	___	___	ELECTRODE IMPEDANCE			___	___	___	___
	REFERENCE	___	___				___	___	___	___
	GROUND	___	___				___	___	___	___

RECORD	EAR	TRANS-DUCER	STIM	RISE	DUR	POLARITY	RATE	LEVEL	# SWEEPS	GAIN	WINDOW	FILTERS
1												
2												
3												
4												
5												
6												
7												
8												
9												
10												
11												
12												
13												
14												
15												
16												
17												
18												
19												
20												
21												

PARAMETERS FOR CLICK THRESHOLDS

CLICK-INSERT EARPHONES

GENERAL SETUP   **AMPLIFIER SETUP**
                                     Channel 1
Test: AEP   Gain: 100000
Channels: 1   Hi Filter: 1500.00
Window: 15.000   Low Filter: 100.00
Pre/Post: 0   Notch filter: out
Points: 256   Artifact: enabled
                        Electrodes: Fz/Ma/Ma

              STIMULUS SETUP
              Stimulator: Insert   Type: rarefacting click   70 dB nHL
              Max # Stim.: 3000
              Rate (/s): 38.0   Ear: right   mask: white 40 dB

CLICK-BONE VIBRATOR

GENERAL SETUP   **AMPLIFIER SETUP**
                                     Channel 1
Test: AEP   Gain: 100000
Channels: 1   Hi Filter: 1500.00
Window: 15.000   Low Filter: 100.00
Pre/Post: 0   Notch filter: out
Points: 256   Artifact: enabled
                        Electrodes: Fz/Ma/Ma

              STIMULUS SETUP
              Stimulator: Bone   Type: rarefacting click   40 dB nHL
              Max # Stim.: 3000
              Rate (/s): 38.0   Ear: left   mask: white 40 dB

PARAMETERS FOR TONEBURST THRESHOLDS

500-Hz tonebursts

GENERAL SETUP   AMPLIFIER SETUP
                          Channel 1
Test: AEP   Gain: 100000
Channels: 1   Hi Filter: 1500
Window: 25.000   Low Filter: 30.00
Pre/Post: 0   Notch filter: out
Points: 256   Artifact: enabled
                          Electrodes: Fz/Ma/Ma

STIMULUS SETUP
Stimulator: Insert
Type:alternating toneburst   50 dB nHL
Max # Stim.: 1500   500 Hz plat: 1.00   rise: 2.0 msec.
Rate (/s): 38.0   Ear: right   mask: white   40 dB

4000/2000/1000-Hz tonebursts

GENERAL SETUP   AMPLIFIER SETUP
                          Channel 1
Test: AEP   Gain: 100000
Channels: 1   Hi Filter: 1500
Window: 15.000   Low Filter: 100.00
Pre/Post: 0   Notch filter: out
Points: 256   Artifact: enabled
                          Electrodes: Fz/Ma/Ma

STIMULUS SETUP
Stimulator: Insert
Type: alternating   tone burst   70 dB nHL
Max # Stim.:   1500   4000 Hz plat: 1.0   rise: 0.5 ms
                      2000 Hz plat: 0.5   rise: 1.0 ms
                      1000 Hz plat: 1.0   rise: 1.0 ms
Rate (/s): 38.0   Ear: right   mask: white   40 dB

THRESHOLD EVALUATION FLOWCHART

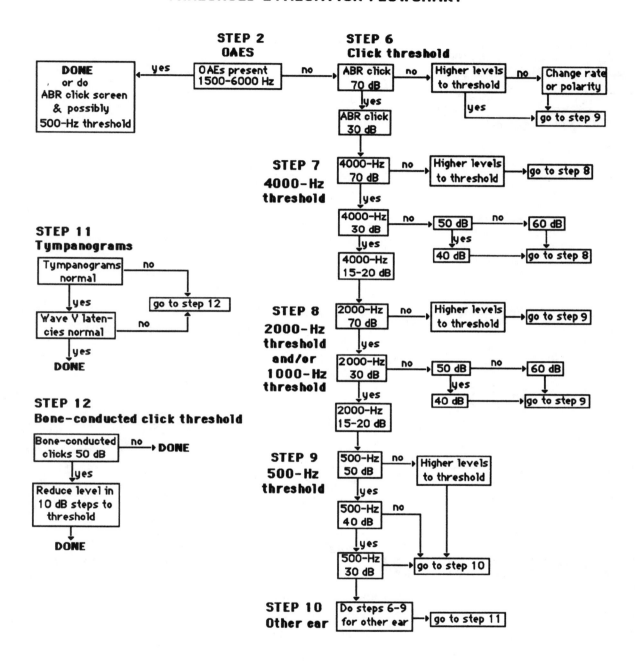

AUDITORY EVOKED POTENTIALS FORM

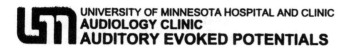

UNIVERSITY OF MINNESOTA HOSPITAL AND CLINIC
AUDIOLOGY CLINIC
AUDITORY EVOKED POTENTIALS

| EXAMINER *J. Hennch* | DATE *8·24·95* | PATIENT BIRTHDATE *7·5·94* |

☒ AUDITORY BRAINSTEM RESPONSE (ABR)
☐ TYMPANIC ELECTROCOCHLEOGRAPHY
☐ TRANSTYMPANIC ELECTROCOCHLEOGRAPHY
☐ INTRAOPERATIVE MONITORING

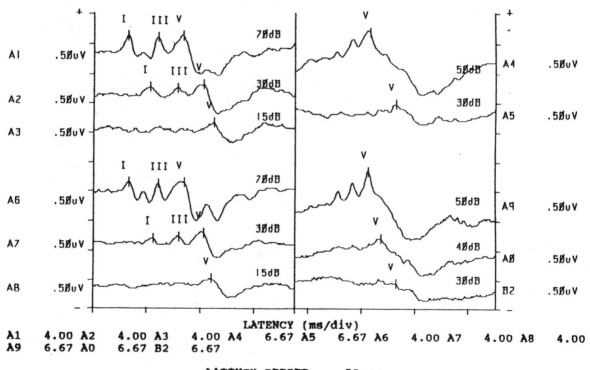

LATENCY (ms/div)

A1 4.00 A2 4.00 A3 4.00 A4 6.67 A5 6.67 A6 4.00 A7 4.00 A8 4.00
A9 6.67 A0 6.67 B2 6.67

LATENCY OFFSET −.80 ms

LATENCIES (ms)

	I	II	III	IV	V	VI	VII	VIII	IX	X
A1	1.78		4.00		5.88					
A2	3.42		5.47		7.40					
A3					8.16					
A4					8.48					
A5					11.70					
A6	1.84		4.00		5.94					
A7	3.65		5.53		7.40					
A8					7.99					
A9					8.28					
A0					9.84					
B2					11.70					

LATENCY/INTENSITY FUNCTION EXAMPLE

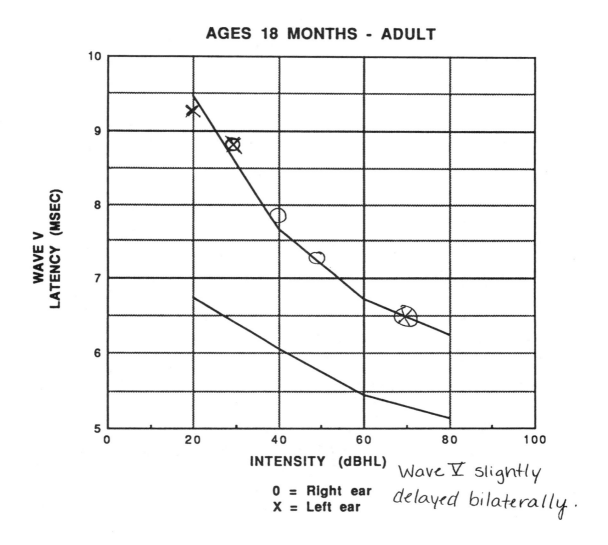

AGES 18 MONTHS - ADULT

0 = **Right ear**
X = **Left ear**

Wave V slightly delayed bilaterally.

AUDITORY BRAINSTEM RESPONSE THRESHOLD EVALUATION

EXAMINER	DATE	BIRTHDATE

ESTIMATED THRESHOLDS

AIR CONDUCTION	500 HZ	1000 HZ	2000 HZ	4000 HZ	CLICKS
Polarity					
Threshold R					
Threshold L					
Reliability					

BONE CONDUCTION	500 HZ	1000 HZ	2000 HZ	4000 HZ	CLICKS
Polarity					
Threshold R					
Threshold L					
Reliability					

WAVE V LATENCIES (See Latency-Intensity Plot)
  RIGHT   ❏ WNL ❏ DELAYED
  LEFT   ❏ WNL ❏ DELAYED
INTERWAVE LATENCIES
  RIGHT   ❏ WNL ❏ DELAYED
  LEFT   ❏ WNL ❏ DELAYED
TYMPANOGRAMS
  RIGHT   ❏ NORMAL ❏ FLAT ❏ ABNORMAL
  LEFT   ❏ NORMAL ❏ FLAT ❏ ABNORMAL
OTOACOUSTIC EMISSIONS
  RIGHT   ❏ PRESENT ❏ ABSENT
  LEFT   ❏ PRESENT ❏ ABSENT

IMPRESSIONS
  RIGHT   ❏ NORMAL HEARING ❏ SENSORINEURAL LOSS ❏ CONDUCTIVE LOSS
  LEFT   ❏ NORMAL HEARING ❏ SENSORINEURAL LOSS ❏ CONDUCTIVE LOSS

COMMENTS

Protocol 15 Infant Hearing Screening

Target Population:
Newborn infants, graduates of the NICU who have predisposing factors which place them at risk for hearing loss, and patients in the Pediatric ICU (see Appendix E and G). A screening might be appropriate for other patients when time constraints prohibit use of the ABR threshold protocol (Protocol 14).

Rationale:
This procedure does not determine thresholds, but attempts to rule out hearing loss, particularly in the 2-4 kHz range. Infant hearing screening enables early identification of hearing loss and facilitates early intervention and secondary prevention.

Equipment Required:
Otoscope
Transient evoked otoacoustic emission system
Acoustic immittance system
Evoked potential system with insert earphones
Surface electrodes
Materials for applying electrodes
        alcohol swabs, skin preparatory materials e.g., NuPrep™ or OMNI-PREP®, gauze pads, scissors, conductive gel or cream (e.g., SYNAPSE®)
Cot or bed

Methods:
1.   Otoscopic inspection. The ear canals should be checked for excessive cerumen (see Protocol 3 Cerumen Removal) and any abnormalities of the ear canal that might affect placement of the otoacoustic emissions infant probe tip or insert earphone.

2.   Transient evoked otoacoustic emission (TEOAE) screen.
        a.   Record TEOAE in a 2.5 -12.5 ms time window with sufficient low frequency filtering to obtain adequate responses from infant ears.
        b.   Select the TEOAE probe tip size and check that the stimulus level is between 80-82 dB SPL and as broad-band and flat as possible in spectrum.
        c.   Adjust the artifact rejection level to 46 dB SPL. If too many responses are being rejected adjust the level to 50 dB SPL.
        d.   Collect at least 100 responses. Fewer responses may be sufficient when the response is readily visible above the noise level and overall reproducibility is greater than 50%.
        e.   Make the determination of pass or fail based on the signal to noise ratios shown on the display. The emission should be at least 3 dB above the noise level at 1.5 kHz and 6 dB above the noise level at 2, 3 and 4 kHz to be considered present in that frequency

band and the emission must be present in three of the four frequency bands to pass the OAE screen.

f.   If the infant fails the initial TEOAE screen, acoustic immittance testing should be performed as soon as possible. For children under four months corrected age, a 226-Hz tympanogram should be obtained first. If it is normal, a 1000-Hz tympanogram and acoustic reflex response using an 1000-Hz probe tone should be obtained. If the immittance testing indicates middle ear problems, a referral to ENT may be appropriate. The TEOAE screen should be repeated after resolution of the middle ear problem. If the immittance testing is normal and both ears fail a second TEOAE screen, the infant should be scheduled for an ABR screen or ABR threshold test, if at risk for progressive loss, as soon as possible.

g.   The patient should be seen for follow-up testing at the time of the NICU 4-month check-up if only one ear fails, or the patient passes but is at risk for progressive hearing loss (see Appendix F). Follow-up testing for progressive hearing loss should proceed as recommended in Appendix G. Also see Appendix I for flowchart for follow-up testing.

3.   ABR Screen.
   a.   Electrode configuration: active: forehead or vertex
                                        reference: ipsilateral mastoid
                                        ground: contralateral mastoid
   b.   Apply electrodes as follows:
         1.   clean skin with alcohol pad
         2.   using a gauze pad moistened with skin preparatory gel, rub skin until it is pink
         3.   apply self-adhesive electrode with a drop of SYNAPSE® placed in the center of the pad; if electrode does not adhere well to the skin, it can be secured with tape.
   c.   Plug the electrodes into the patient connection box and measure electrode impedances. Electrode impedances should be ≤ 3 kohms but sometimes it may be necessary to proceed with electrode impedances ≤ 7 kohms. Record the impedances on the ABR/ECOG Worksheet (see Protocol 14 Appendix A).
   d.   Select appropriate stimulus and data collection parameters. See Appendix B for example of set-up parameters.
   e.   Hearing will be screened using 70 and 30 dB nHL clicks presented at 38/s. Collect one response at 70 dB and if the waves are easily identifiable, collect two responses at 30 dB. Collection of responses for an ear is completed if replicable responses are seen at 30 dB and all waves or at least the most apparent wave (either wave III or wave V) have shifted appropriately relative to the response at 70 dB. Appendix D is an example of Wave V age-related latency-intensity norms (from Gorga et al., 1987). (Note the latency printout and the latency-intensity norms are both corrected by 0.8 ms for the sound tube delay). If the Wave V latencies are outside the normal range, immittance measures should be completed to evaluate for middle ear pathology (see 2f). If no response or a questionable response is seen at 70 dB, increase the intensity 10 to 20 dB to better identify waves.
   f.   Repeat Step 6 for the other ear, starting at 30 dB nHL.
   g.   The following suggestions may help to obtain good and replicable responses.
         1.   For noisy records, try to make the infant more comfortable.
         2.   Average more sweeps.

3.   If a high proportion of responses are being rejected by the artifact reject system, it maybe necessary to reduce the amplifier gain or raise the artifact reject threshold.

4.   If there is any doubt about the presence of a response, do a silent control (-5 dB HL) to determine the noise level.

5.   After checking with a nurse, shut off monitoring equipment and/or isolette (unplug from the wall); remove cables from around the infant.

h.   If either or both ears fail the ABR screening at 30 dB nHL, middle ear problems should be ruled out as in Step 2f with TEOAE screening at 4 months. If either ear fails at 70 dB nHL, follow-up should be completed at an earlier date than the 4-month NICU follow-up visit. If a child is at risk for progressive hearing loss, follow-up testing should proceed as recommended in Appendix G.

Report Format:
TEOAE SCREEN:
Print the octave band analysis for each ear (see Appendix A).

ABR SCREEN:
Patient identification, waveforms, and latencies should be printed out on the Auditory Evoked Potentials Form (see Appendix C). Waveforms should be labeled as to ear stimulated, intensity and repetition rate used. Any changes from standard protocol must also be recorded on the form as well as any other information that may be useful in interpretation may be added.

The TEOAE print-outs or the ABR form, as well as a written chart note of the test results, should be entered into the patient's hospital chart. A letter explaining the results of this test, along with a brochure that discusses normal hearing and speech development, should be given to the parents. The following 3 types of letters can be seen in Appendix H:
1.   Pass screening - no progressive loss suspected
2.   Pass screening - progressive loss possible
3.   Fail screening

Information should be entered into the NICU database for follow-up purposes.

Billing:
Bill Otoacoustic Emission (CPT 92587); 1 unit for each 15 minute unit of patient contact time.
Bill Immittance Testing (CPT 92567).
Bill Auditory Brainstem Response (CPT 92585 or CPT 92599 if sedated); 1 unit for each 15-minute unit of patient contact time.

References:
Cox, L. C. (1985). Infant assessment: Developmental and age-related considerations. In J. T. Jacobson (Ed.), *The Auditory Brainstem Response* (pp. 297-316). San Diego: College-Hill Press.

Gorga, M. P., Reiland, J. K., Beauchane, K. A., Worthington, D. W., & Jesteadt, W. (1987). Auditory brainstem responses from graduates of an intensive care nursery: Normal patterns of response. *Journal of Speech and Hearing Research, 30*, 311-318.

Hall, J. W. III. (1992). *Handbook of Auditory Evoked Potentials.* Boston: Allyn & Bacon.

Kemp, D. T., & Ryan, S. (1991). Otoacoustic emission tests in neonatal screening programmes. *Acta Otolaryngologica (Stockholm)*, (Supplement 482), 73-84.

Norton, S. J. (1994). Emerging role of evoked otoacoustic emissions in neonatal hearing screening. *American Journal of Otology, 15* (Supplement 1), 4-12.

Schwartz, D. M., & Schwartz, J. A. (1991). Auditory evoked potentials in clinical pediatrics. In W. F. Rintelmann (Ed.), *Hearing Assessment* (pp. 429-476). Austin, TX: Pro-Ed.

Protocol 15 Appendix

A.   Transient Evoked Otoacoustic Emissions Analysis-Print Out
B.   Parameter Example: Clicks (Insert Phones)
C.   Auditory Evoked Potentials Example
D.   Norms for Age-Related Wave V Latencies by Intensity
E.   Risk Criteria for Neonates and Infants
F.   Criteria for Follow-Up
G.   Predisposing Factors for Hearing Loss
H.   Sample Letters for Parents
I.   Infant Hearing Screening Flowchart

TRANSIENT EVOKED OTOACOUSTIC EMISSIONS ANALYSIS EXAMPLE

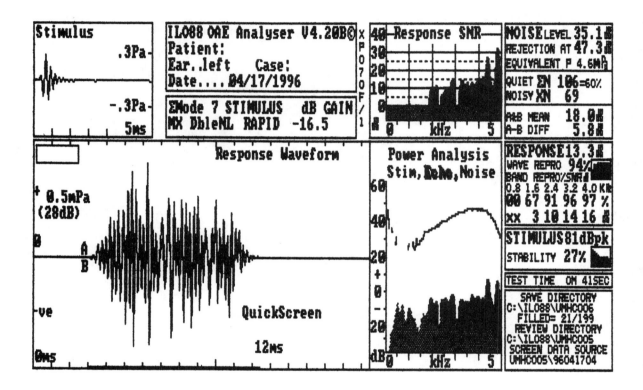

PARAMETER EXAMPLE: CLICKS (INSERT PHONES)

Collection Parameters

GENERAL SETUP   AMP SETUP
                              Channel 1
Test: AEP   Gain: 100000
Channel: 1   Hi filter: 1500.00
Window: 15.000   Low filter: 30.00
pre/post: 0   Notch filter: out
Points: 256   Artifact: enabled
                              Electrode: fz/ma/ma

STIMULUS SETUP

dB   Stimulator: insert   tYpe: rarefaction click 70

                        Max # stim: 3000
                        Rate (/s):   38/s   Ear: left   mask: none

Comments:

AUDITORY BRAINSTEM RESPONSE WAVEFORM EXAMPLE

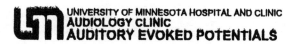

UNIVERSITY OF MINNESOTA HOSPITAL AND CLINIC
AUDIOLOGY CLINIC
AUDITORY EVOKED POTENTIALS

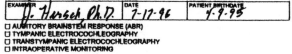

☐ AUDITORY BRAINSTEM RESPONSE (ABR)
☐ TYMPANIC ELECTROCOCHLEOGRAPHY
☐ TRANSTYMPANIC ELECTROCOCHLEOGRAPHY
☐ INTRAOPERATIVE MONITORING

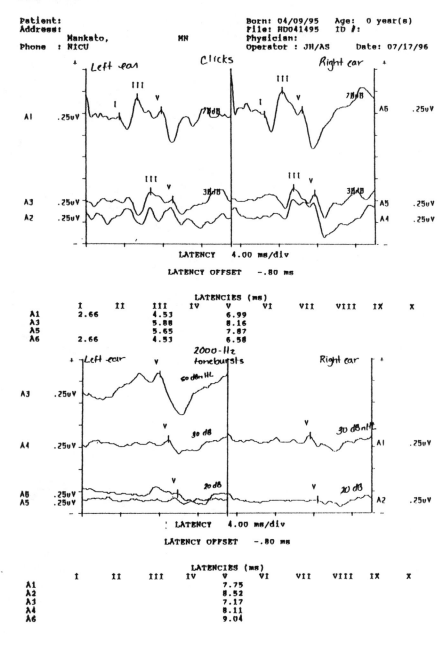

NORMS FOR AGE-RELATED WAVE V LATENCIES BY INTENSITY
(from Gorga et al., 1987)

Ages 33-36 weeks

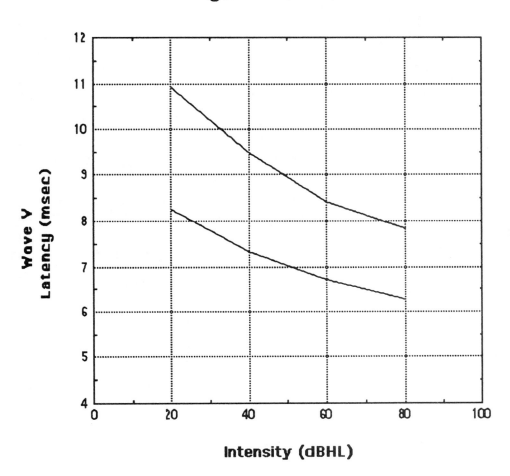

NORMS FOR AGE-RELATED WAVE V LATENCIES BY INTENSITY
(from Gorga et al., 1987)

Ages 37-40 weeks

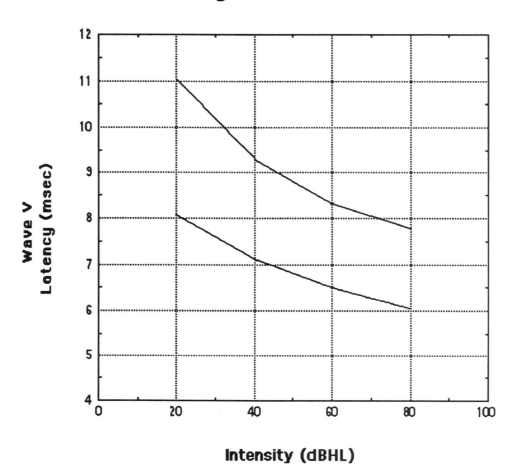

Intensity (dBHL)

NORMS FOR AGE-RELATED WAVE V LATENCIES BY INTENSITY
(from Gorga et al., 1987)

Ages 41-44 Weeks

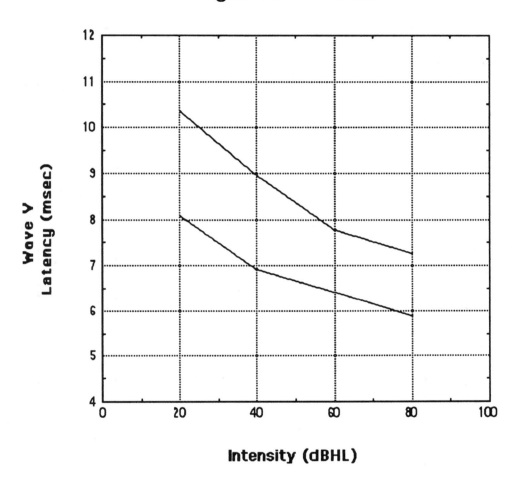

NORMS FOR AGE-RELATED WAVE V LATENCIES BY INTENSITY
(from Gorga et al., 1987)

Ages 3-9 months

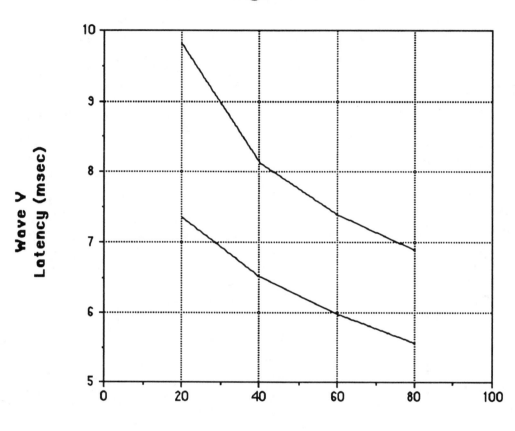

Intensity (dBHL)

NORMS FOR AGE-RELATED WAVE V LATENCIES BY INTENSITY
(from Gorga et al., 1987)

Ages 9-18 months

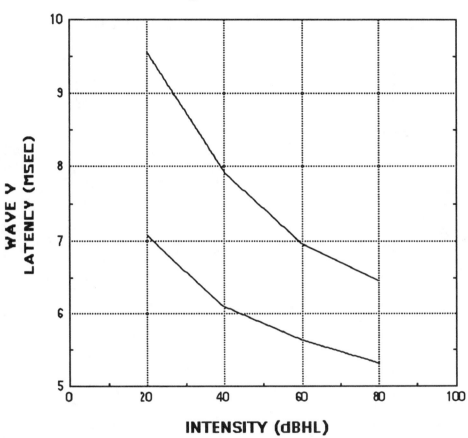

NORMS FOR AGE-RELATED WAVE V LATENCIES BY INTENSITY
(from Gorga et al., 1987)

Ages 18 months – adult

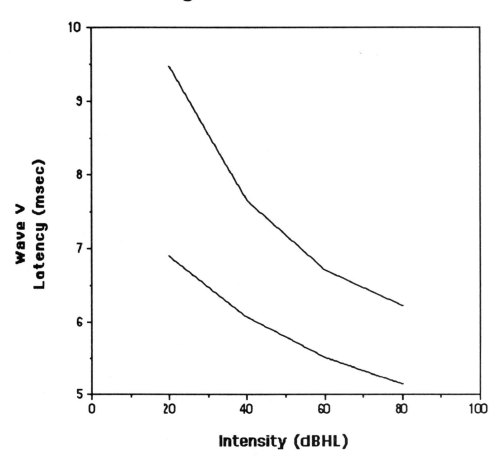

RISK CRITERIA FOR NEONATES AND INFANTS

RISK CRITERIA: NEONATES (BIRTH-28 DAYS)

1.   Family history hereditary childhood sensorineural hearing loss.

2.   In utero infection, such as cytomegalovirus, rubella, syphilis, herpes, and toxoplasmosis.

3.   Craniofacial anomalies including those with morphologic abnormalities of the pinna and ear canal.

4.   Birth weight less than 1,500 grams (about 3.3 lbs).

5.   Hyperbilirubinemia at a serum level requiring exchange transfusion.

6.   Ototoxic medications including but not limited to the aminoglycosides, used in multiple courses or in combination with loop diuretics.

7.   Bacterial meningitis.

8.   Apgar scores of 0-4 at 1 minute or 0-6 at 5 minutes.

9.   Mechanical ventilation lasting 5 days or longer.

10.   Stigmata or other findings associated with a syndrome known to include a sensorineural and/or conductive hearing loss.

RISK CRITERIA: INFANTS (29 days - 2 years) when certain health conditions develop that require rescreening.

The factors that identify those infants who are at-risk for sensorineural hearing impairment include the following:

1.   Parent/caregiver concern regarding hearing, speech, language and/or developmental delay.

2.   Bacterial meningitis and other infections associated with sensorineural hearing loss.

3.   Hear trauma associated with loss of consciousness or skull fracture.

4.   Stigmata or other findings associated with syndromes known to include a sensorineural and/or conductive hearing loss.

5.   Ototoxic medications, including but not limited to chemotherapeutic agents or aminoglycosides, used in multiple courses or in combination with loop diuretics.

6.   Recurrent or persistent otitis media with effusion for at least 3 months.

RISK CRITERIA FOR NEONATES AND INFANTS *page 2*

Risk Criteria: Infants (29 days - 3 years) who require periodic monitoring of hearing

Some newborns and infants may pass initial hearing screening but require periodic monitoring of hearing to detect delayed-onset sensorineural and/or conductive hearing loss. Infants with these indicators require hearing evaluation at least every 6 months until age 3 years, and at appropriate intervals thereafter.

Indicators associated with delayed onset sensorineural hearing loss include:
1.   Family history of hereditary childhood hearing loss.

2.   In utero infection, such as cytomegalovirus, rubella, syphilis, herpes, or toxoplasmosis.

3.   Neurofibromatosis Type II and neurodegenerative disorders.

Indicators associated with conductive hearing loss include:

1.   Recurrent or persistent otitis media with effusion.

2.   Anatomic deformities and other disorders that affect eustachian tube function.

3.   Neurodegenerative disorders.

Joint Committee on Infant Hearing. (1994). 1994 Position statement. *Asha, 36*, 38-41.

CRITERIA FOR FOLLOW-UP OF INFANTS PASSING INITIAL SCREEN

1.   Persistent pulmonary hypertension requiring hyperventilation with a ph > 7.55 for 12 hours or more.

2.   Significant exposure to ototoxic drugs

    a.   Concurrent use of two ototoxic drugs for more than 7 days (most likely lasix/ gentamicin).

    b.   Use of one or more ototoxic drugs during periods of renal failure (creatinine $\geq$ 1.4 suggested).

    c.   Abnormally high level of ototoxic drug for $\geq$ 3 days.

3.   TORCH infection.

4.   CHARGE Syndrome

5.   Family history of hearing loss.

6.   Bacterial meningitis.

7.   At the time of the NICU Clinic appointment, if the parents or clinic staff are concerned about the infant's hearing, the infant should be tested.

It is recommended that infants falling into these groups be retested at the same time as the 4-month (corrected age) NICU follow-up clinic visit. All follow-up hearing tests should be ordered at discharge as Acoustic Immittance/Otoacoustic Emission testing.

See Appendix G for information regarding the appropriate monitoring schedule, after the 4 month appointment, based on risk factor.

Consultation with the attending neonatologist is suggested if there is any uncertainty whether the infant falls into any of the groups listed above.

PREDISPOSING FACTORS FOR HEARING LOSS

DEFECTS OF THE HEAD AND NECK: anomalies associated with craniofacial and skeletal syndromes: (also take note if there are renal anomalies).
Cleft lip and/or palate and external ear anomalies (e.g., malformed pinnas, low set ears, ear tags) may be associated with middle ear anomalies in either ear.   Ear malformations may also be associated with certain renal disorders.

Hearing loss is conductive with cleft lip and palate and most external ear anomalies.
Hearing loss may be varied in type and severity when the anomalies are associated with syndromes.
Not normally progressive.

LOW BIRTHWEIGHT (less than 1500 grams):   this in itself may not be the causal factor for a hearing loss--hearing loss may be associated with related problems i.e.. anoxia, hyperbilirubinemia, increased incidence of bacterial and viral infections, treatment with ototoxic drugs.

Hearing loss is generally sensorineural, high frequency and steeply sloping.   There is also a high correlation between birthweight and otitis media, especially with prolonged ventilation.
Not normally progressive: be aware of treatments used, however.

HYPERBILIRUBINEMIA: excessive amounts of bilirubin in the blood can be neurotoxic.
If the bilirubin is not detoxified by the liver, in severe cases it may cross the blood/brain barrier (kernicterus).

Hearing loss is usually sensorineural, mild to profound, bilateral or unilateral.
Not normally progressive.

FAMILY HISTORY: hereditary hearing impairment.

Hearing loss may be any type and degree depending on the syndrome or hereditary condition.
May be PROGRESSIVE or late-onset hearing loss: monitoring is dependent on the hereditary condition.

BACTERIAL MENINGITIS: infection of the meninges (*in utero* or during delivery).
The meningitis infection may pass to the inner ear via the cochlear aqueduct or the internal auditory meatus.   Hearing loss may also be secondary to the treatment of meningitis with ototoxic drugs i.e. Kanamycin and Gentamicin.

Hearing loss is often a severe-profound sensorineural loss bilaterally, however, it may be milder, unilateral and sometimes progressive. (There are some documented cases of improvement, also.)
Possibly PROGRESSIVE: monitor for the first year.

PREDISPOSING FACTORS FOR HEARING LOSS *page 2*

CONGENITAL (prior to intra-partum)/PERINATAL (shortly before or after birth) INFECTIONS (TORCH COMPLEX):

TOXOPLASMOSIS: infection from parasite Toxoplasma gondii (sometimes from uncooked meat or contact with cat feces). There are changes in the soft tissue mesenchyme, mucoperiosteum, and calcium deposits in the spiral ligament (mainly stria vascularis) of the inner ear.

> Hearing loss is often moderate to profound sensorineural.
> Possibly PROGRESSIVE: monitor for the first year or until normal speech develops.

SYPHILIS: sexually transmitted bacterial infection in adults which is then transmitted to child *in utero*.

> Hearing loss is often a sudden sensorineural hearing loss--profound and bilateral.
> Poor word recognition abilities have been observed because of neural atrophy.
> Possibly PROGRESSIVE: monitor every six months until 2 years old, intermittently after.

RUBELLA: airborne transmitted disease contracted by the mother, which can then enter the embryo; it is particularly a problem if the mother is infected during the 1st trimester.

> Hearing loss is often severe-to-profound sensorineural -"cookie-bite" in the mid-frequency range.
> May be PROGRESSIVE or very late onset: monitor hearing for at least two years.

CYTOMEGALOVIRUS: transmitted perinatally or postnatally
Problems: enlarged liver, spleen, jaundice, chorioretinitis, cerebral calcification and microcephaly-if severe, may manifest global CNS infections involving the cerebral cortex, brainstem, cochlear nuclei, as well as the cranial nerves and inner ear. Hearing loss can also be present with asymptomatic CMV (reports suggest 17-55%).

> Hearing loss ranges from mild to profound sensorineural impairments: bilateral or unilateral.
> Possibly PROGRESSIVE virus may remain active for several years: monitor every 3 months for first year and continue monitoring until normal speech develops.

HERPES SIMPLEX VIRUS: sexually transmitted virus with transmission to the infant during the birthing process-may result in death with only 4% surviving without sequelae. The virus may infect the sensory cells of the labyrinth.

> Hearing loss probably sensorineural - degree not well documented.
> Possibly PROGRESSIVE--not well documented.

CHARGE SYNDROME: A syndrome with multiple congenital anomalies, with the mnemonic "CHARGE" being used to describe the most common anomalies: Coloboma of the eye, Heart disease, Atresia of the choanae, Retarded growth, development and/or CNS anomalies, Genital hypoplasia, and Ear anomalies and/or deafness.

PREDISPOSING FACTORS FOR HEARING LOSS *page 3*

Hearing loss is, in most cases, a moderately-severe, mixed loss with a "wedge" or peak shaped audiogram (losses range from mild to profound). Typically, the loss is conductive in the low frequencies (due to ossicular anomalies and/or middle ear effusion) and sensorineural in the high frequencies.

Both the conductive and sensorineural components may be PROGRESSIVE: monitor closely during first year of life, then on an annual basis after age one.

OTOTOXICITY: (aminoglycoside and/or diuretic therapy)

Child is more at risk if there are simultaneous treatments of two or more ototoxic drugs, prolonged duration of treatment, or renal impairment during treatment.

Hearing loss is often a high frequency sensorineural loss (may be a flat sensorineural hearing loss with diuretics).

Possibly PROGRESSIVE: monitor several months after treatment is discontinued.

PROLONGED MECHANICAL VENTILATION: (e.g., Persistent Pulmonary Hypertension-sometimes referred to as Persistent Fetal Circulation)

With increased oxygen, the body's autoregulation system may decrease blood flow-so less glucose and nutrients are transported throughout the body. This may affect cell metabolism. Outer Hair Cells are often the first part of the cochlea to be affected.

Hearing loss is often a high frequency sensorineural loss.

Possibly PROGRESSIVE more often observed when ventilated for 10 days or more: monitor for several months after ventilation is discontinued.

References:

Gerkin, K. P. (1984). The high risk register for deafness. *Asha, 26*, 17-23.

Kasanoff, J. L., & Gist, K. (1989). Progressive sensorineural hearing loss in NICU graduates: Follow-up recommendations. *Asha, 31*, 112.

Pettigrew, A., Edwards, D., & Henderson-Smart, D. (1988). Perinatal risk factors in preterm infants with moderate to severe hearing deficits. *Medical Journal of Australia, 148*, 174-177.

Phelps, O. L. (1982). Neonatal oxygen toxicity: Is it preventable?. *The Pediatric Clinic of North America: The Newborn.*

Quick, C. (1980). Chemical and drug effects in the inner ear. In M. Paparella & D. Shumrick (Eds.), *Otolaryngology*: Vol. II (pp. 1804-1824). W.B. Saunders Co.

Rosenhall, U., & Kankkunen, A. (1980). Hearing alterations following meningitis. *Ear and Hearing, 1*, 185-190.

Thelin, J. W., Mitchell, J. A., Hefner, M. A., & Davenport, S. L. H., (1986). CHARGE Syndrome. Part II. Hearing loss. *International Journal of Pediatric Otorhinolaryngology, 12*, 145-163.

SAMPLE LETTERS FOR PARENTS

Pass NICU Screening

Dear Parents:

Your child passed the hearing screening test before leaving the hospital. This test screens the hearing system's responses to clicks (high pitched sounds). Passing this screening test means that your child probably hears important speech sounds in each ear and his/her hearing should not prevent speech development. However, it is not a guarantee that your child will continue to hear normally.

It is important that if your child is not talking at appropriate age levels (see attached brochure) you should consult your family physician and consider a hearing evaluation by an audiologist. Please be aware that the ages on the brochure should be corrected by how many months your child was premature. Also, please feel free to contact the Audiology Clinic if you have any questions.

Pass NICU screening: progressive loss

Dear Parents:

Your child passed the hearing screening test before leaving the hospital. This test screens the hearing system's responses to clicks (high pitched sounds). Passing the screening test means that, at this time, your child probably hears the important speech sounds in each ear.

However, your child has a pre-existing condition which may result in changes in hearing. Consequently, it is recommended that your child's hearing be rechecked at the time of the NICU follow-up visit. Please feel free to contact the Audiology Clinic if you have any questions.

Fail NICU screening

Dear Parents:

Your child did not pass the hearing screening test before leaving the hospital. This test screens the hearing system's responses to clicks (high-pitched sounds). Since this is a screening test, it does not necessarily mean your child has a permanent hearing impairment. However, it is important that your child's hearing be thoroughly investigated, as good hearing is essential to the development of speech and language skills.

Your child should return for a hearing recheck at the time of the NICU follow-up visit. Please feel free to contact the Audiology Clinic if you have any questions.

INFANT HEARING SCREENING FLOW CHART

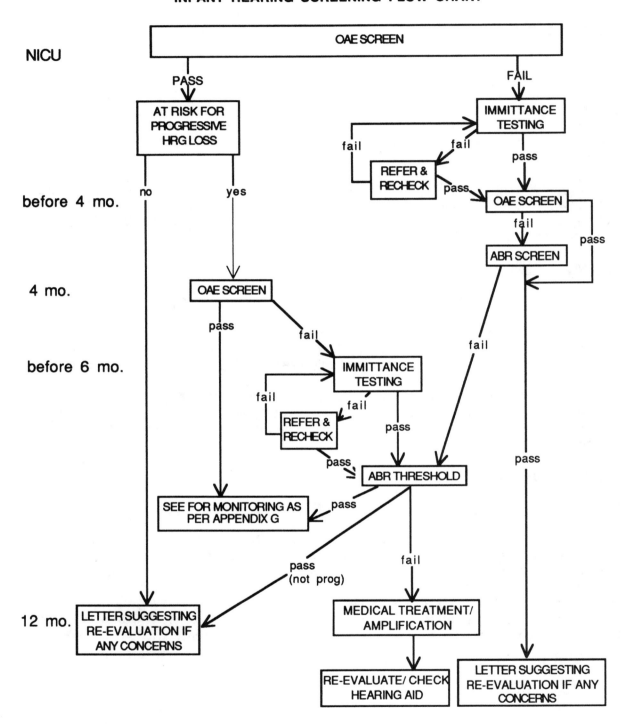

Protocol 16
Tympanic Electrocochleography (ECOG)

Target Population:

1. Patients who are at risk for endolymphatic hydrops. Symptoms include fluctuating hearing loss, often asymmetrical; unilateral or bilateral fluctuating tinnitus; sensation of fullness in the ear; episodic vertigo. The hearing loss in early stages of hydrops is sensorineural, often more severe in the low frequencies. The results are most diagnostic when the patient is most symptomatic and in early stages of the disease.

2. ECOG may be performed as part of the preoperative evaluation of patients scheduled for surgery with intraoperative auditory monitoring.

Rationale:

ECOG results are useful for distinguishing between hearing losses related to endolymphatic hydrops and sensorineural hearing loss caused by non-hydropic processes. Abnormalities may take the form of an increased summating potential/compound action potential (SP/AP) ratio, a latency difference between action potentials elicited by condensation and rarefaction clicks, an increased summating potential to a tone burst, or other abnormalities in AP morphology. ECOG is one of the few functional tests for endolymphatic hydrops. The outcome of this evaluation may influence medical and/or surgical management.

Because many patients who are at risk for endolymphatic hydrops are also at risk for VIII Nerve disease, auditory brainstem response (ABR) is usually performed simultaneously with ECOG.

Equipment Required:
Surgical microscope
Nasal speculum
0.9% saline
Electrode cream (e.g. SYNAPSE®)
Alcohol pads
Conductive abrasive (e.g., Nu-Prep™ or OMNI-PREP®)
Disposable surface electrodes
Tympanic membrane wick electrode
Evoked potential recording system with shielded insert earphone
Elevated bed

Methods:

1. <u>Otoscopic Inspection</u>. The ear canals will be inspected otoscopically to rule out excessive cerumen and active ear disease. Excessive cerumen should be removed (Protocol 3). When active disease is suspected, a physician will be consulted before proceeding with the evaluation.

2.   <u>Apply a Surface Electrode to the High Forehead Area and Each Mastoid.</u>
        a.   Clean skin with alcohol pad.
        b.   Using a gauze pad moistened with abrasive solution, rub skin until it is pink.
        c.   Apply electrode insuring that it adheres well to the skin. If it does not, it can be
        secured with tape.

3.   <u>Preparation and Placement of the Tympanic Membrane Wick Electrode</u>. The wick is
saturated in 0.9% saline mixed with a drop of electrode cream. Upon removal from the saline
mixture, the wick is trimmed to a diameter of 2-4 mm depending on the size of the patient's
ear. The electrode should be placed with direct visualization aided by an operating microscope.
Holding the placement shaft, the electrode is lowered until it is observed to contact the eardrum,
preferably on the umbo. The electrode shaft is placed in the tragal notch.

4.   <u>Place Ear Insert</u>. A foam ear insert coupled to the insert earphone is inserted in the ear
canal. It is squeezed to the smallest possible diameter and inserted alongside the electrode lead.
The pediatric size foam insert is best for most patients.

Caution - Turn equipment power on before connecting patient.

5.   <u>Connect Electrode Cables As Follows</u>:
        Channel 1 Active - forehead
        Channel 1 Reference - ipsilateral mastoid
        Channel 2 Active - tympanic membrane
        Channel 2 Reference - forehead
        Ground - Contralateral mastoid
With this configuration, Channel 1 is set up for ABR and Channel 2 for ECOG.

6.   <u>Check Electrode Impedances</u>. Surface electrode impedances should be $\leq$ 5 kohm. The wick
electrode impedance should be < 70 kohm, although good quality recordings are sometimes
obtained with much higher impedances. Higher impedances result in larger stimulus artifacts.
Impedances are recorded on the ECOG/ABR Worksheet (see Protocol 14, Appendix A).

7.   <u>Evoked Potential Recording</u>. Recording parameters are presented in Appendix A,
ECOG/ABR Click Setup. Click evoked potentials are recorded to condensation and rarefaction
clicks. If they are recorded in separate trials, an alternating polarity condition may also be
recorded. If condensation and rarefaction conditions are recorded concurrently, the responses
can be averaged to obtain the alternating polarity response. 1000 repetitions of each polarity
per run are collected unless the recordings are unusually noisy, requiring more repetitions. A
repetition of the first run frequently produces a better quality recording as the patient becomes
relaxed. Use contralateral masking as appropriate.

ABR is collected concurrently in another channel of the evoked potential system.

Tone burst responses are obtained to 1-kHz and 2-kHz tones (rise-fall = 5.0 ms; plateau = 5.0
ms). See Appendix A for example of ECOG/ABR Tone Setup. The summating potential amplitude
is measured from the midpoint between a positive and negative peak during a stable portion of
the response, typically 6-8 ms, to a moving baseline created by connecting the baseline at onset
of the cochlear microphonic with the baseline at offset (see Appendix C).

Stimulus and recording parameters for each trial are recorded on the ECOG/ABR Worksheet.

8.   Interpretation. Any of the following is suggestive of endolymphatic hydrops:
        a.   in the alternating click response, the SP/AP ratio exceeds 0.43,
        b.   the difference in AP latency for condensation and rarefaction clicks exceeds 0.38 ms.,
        c.   a summating potential on the tone burst response more negative than 1.75 µV at 1 kHz and 2.25 µV at 2 kHz.

Report Format:

The results are summarized in a chart note and ECOG results are plotted on the Auditory Evoked Potentials Form (see Appendices B-D). The responses are labelled with the stimulus type, polarity, and level.

Billing:

Bill Electrocochleography (CPT 92584); one or two 15-minute units
Bill Auditory Brainstem Response (CPT 92585); one 15-minute unit.

References:

Eggermont, J. J. (1976). Electrocochleography. In W. D. Keidel & W. D. Neff (Eds.), *Handbook of Sensory Physiology,* Volume 5/3 (pp. 626-705). Springer Verlag, Berlin.

Levine, S. C., Margolis, R. H., Fournier, E. M., & Winzenburg, S. M. (1992). Tympanic electrocochleography for evaluation of endolymphatic hydrops. *Laryngoscope, 102,* 614-622.

Margolis, R. H. (1996). Electrocochleography. *Seminars in Hearing, in press.*

Margolis, R. H., Levine, S. C., Fournier, E. M., Hunter, L. L., Smith, S. L., & Lilly, D. J. (1992). Tympanic electrocochleography: Normal and abnormal patterns of response. *Audiology, 31,* 8-24.

Margolis, R. H., Rieks, D., Fournier, E. M., & Levine, S. E. (1995). Tympanic electrocochleography for diagnosis of Ménière's disease. *Achieves Otolaryngology Head Neck Surgery, 121,* 44-55.

Ruth, R. A. (1994). Electrocochleography. In J. Katz (Ed.), *Handbook of Clinical Audiology* (pp. 339-350). Baltimore: Williams & Wilkins

Protocol 16 Appendix

A.   Parameter Setup
B.   Electrocochleography Waveform Example Showing Click Responses
C.   Electrocochleography Waveform Example Showing Tone Burst Responses
D.   Auditory Evoked Potentials Example Showing Auditory Brainstem Response
E.   Example of Electrocochleography Report

PARAMETER SETUP

ECOG/ABR CLICK SETUP

GENERAL SETUP   AMPLIFIER SETUP

		Channel 1	Channel 2
Test: P300	Gain:	100000	100000
Channels: 2	Hi Filter:	3000	3000
Window: 10.000	Low Filter:	100	3
Pre/Post: 0	Notch filter:	out	out
Points: 256	Artifact:	enabled	disabled
	Electrodes:	Fz/Ma/Ma	TM/Fz/Ma

STIMULUS SETUP

Stimulator:	Insert	Type: condensing click	88 dB nHL
Max # Stim.:	1000		
Rate (/s):	13.0	Ear: right mask: white	40 dB eff. mask. level
P300 ratio:	1		
		infrequent stim: rarefacting click	88 dB nHL

ECOG/ABR TONE SETUP

GENERAL SETUP   AMPLIFIER SETUP

		Channel 1	Channel 2
Test: P300	Gain:	100000	100000
Channels: 2	Hi Filter:	3000	3000
Window: 20.000	Low Filter:	100	3
Pre/Post: 0	Notch filter:	out	out
Points: 256	Artifact:	enabled	disabled
	Electrodes:	Fz/Ma/Ma	TM/Fz/Ma

STIMULUS SETUP

Stimulator:	Insert	Type: condensing tone burst	110 dB SPL
Max # Stim.:	1000	1000 Hz plat: 5.0 ms	rise 5.0 ms
Rate (/s):	38.0	Ear: right mask: white	40 dB eff. mask. level
P300 ratio:	1		
		infrequent stim: rarefacting tone burst	110 dB SPL

ELECTROCOCHLEOGRAPHY WAVEFORM EXAMPLE
SHOWING CLICK RESPONSES

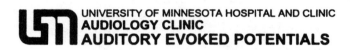

UNIVERSITY OF MINNESOTA HOSPITAL AND CLINIC
AUDIOLOGY CLINIC
AUDITORY EVOKED POTENTIALS

EXAMINER R. Macylin	DATE 6-12-96	PATIENT BIRTHDATE 11-19-52

☐ AUDITORY BRAINSTEM RESPONSE (ABR)
☒ TYMPANIC ELECTROCOCHLEOGRAPHY
☐ TRANSTYMPANIC ELECTROCOCHLEOGRAPHY
☐ INTRAOPERATIVE MONITORING

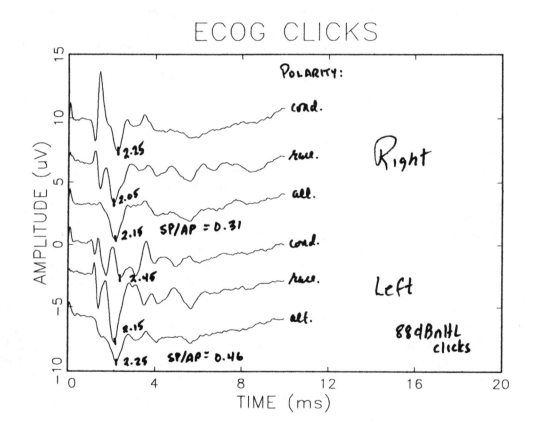

ELECTROCOCHLEOGRAPHY WAVEFORM EXAMPLE
SHOWING TONE BURST RESPONSES

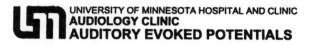

UNIVERSITY OF MINNESOTA HOSPITAL AND CLINIC
AUDIOLOGY CLINIC
AUDITORY EVOKED POTENTIALS

EXAMINER R. Macedie	DATE 6-12-96	PATIENT BIRTHDATE 11-19-52

☐ AUDITORY BRAINSTEM RESPONSE (ABR)
☒ TYMPANIC ELECTROCOCHLEOGRAPHY
☐ TRANSTYMPANIC ELECTROCOCHLEOGRAPHY
☐ INTRAOPERATIVE MONITORING

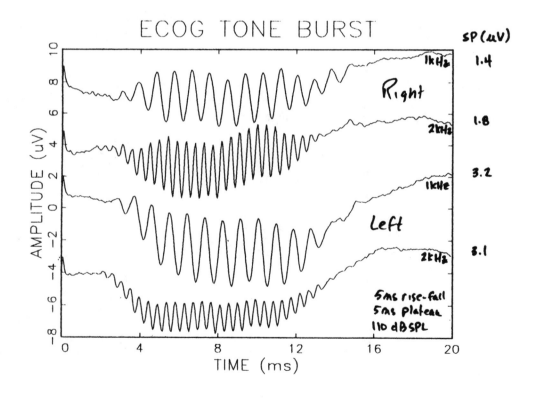

AUDITORY EVOKED POTENTIALS EXAMPLE
SHOWING AUDITORY BRAINSTEM RESPONSE

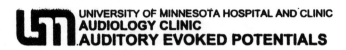

UNIVERSITY OF MINNESOTA HOSPITAL AND CLINIC
AUDIOLOGY CLINIC
AUDITORY EVOKED POTENTIALS

| EXAMINER R. Macydis | DATE 6-12-96 | PATIENT BIRTHDATE 11-19-52 |

☑ AUDITORY BRAINSTEM RESPONSE (ABR)
☐ TYMPANIC ELECTROCOCHLEOGRAPHY
☐ TRANSTYMPANIC ELECTROCOCHLEOGRAPHY
☐ INTRAOPERATIVE MONITORING

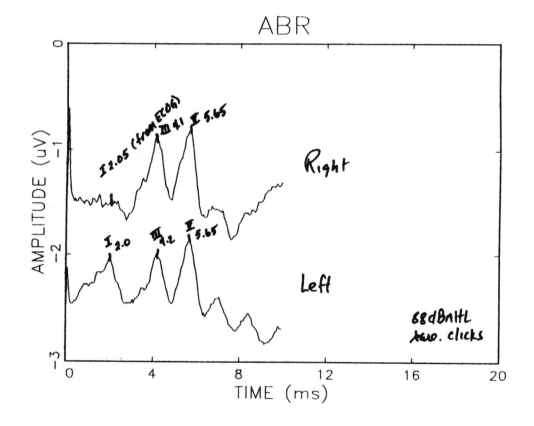

EXAMPLE OF ELECTROCOCHLEOGRAPHY REPORT

Electrocochleography   Evaluation

BACKGROUND:

This 43-year old female patient was referred by Dr.   for tympanic electrocochleography (ECOG) to evaluate the possibility of endolymphatic hydrops and for auditory brainstem response (ABR) to evaluate retrocochlear function. Two months ago during an upper respiratory infection she noticed a drop in hearing in the left ear. At that time (4-30-96) she had a mild low frequency sensorineural loss and a moderate high frequency loss with normal hearing in the mid frequencies. Her hearing was improved on 5-14-96. On 6-11-96 it had dropped to a 50 dB flat sensorineural loss with poor word recognition. She has had aural fullness and tinnitus in the left ear with no vestibular symptoms.

PROCEDURES AND RESULTS:

Tympanic electrocochleography (ECOG) was performed with an electrode on each tympanic membrane. Click and tone burst responses were normal in the right ear. Click and tone burst responses from the left ear were characterized by abnormal summating potentials.

ABR was recorded from scalp electrodes with 88-dB nHL rarefaction click stimuli presented to each ear. ABR responses were normal and bilaterally symmetrical.

SUMMARY/RECOMMENDATIONS:

ECOG responses suggest cochlear hydrops in the left ear. ABR responses do not suggest disease of the auditory pathway.

Audiologist

Protocol 17 Intraoperative Auditory Monitoring

Target Population:

Patients undergoing surgery that places the auditory system at risk and patients undergoing procedures for relief of endolymphatic hydrops. These include hearing preservation procedures for removal of acoustic neuromas, vestibular nerve sections, nerve decompression procedures, and endolymphatic sac procedures.

Rationale:

In procedures that place the auditory system at risk, intraoperative auditory monitoring provides feedback to the surgeon regarding the status of auditory function that can be useful in preserving hearing. In endolymphatic sac procedures for patients with abnormal electrocochleograms (ECOG), intraoperative monitoring may be useful for detecting changes in cochlear function. Intraoperative auditory monitoring is performed by measuring the compound action potential (AP) by transtympanic electrocochleography. In addition, the cochlear microphonic (CM), summating potential (SP), and auditory brainstem response (ABR) may be monitored.

Equipment Required:

Portable evoked potential equipment
Transtympanic needle electrodes (12 mm or 75 mm stainless steel electrodes can be used.
    Insulated electrodes are preferable)
Electrode impedance meter (battery powered)
Oscilloscope, probe microphone preamplifier, microphone/cable assembly
Disposable foam ear insert with probe microphone tube inserted
Shielded Insert earphones (Etymotic Research ER-3A) with modified sound delivery tube
VCR and monitor screen
Video cable
Mini jumper cable
Nasal speculum
Alligator forceps (for inserting 12 mm electrode)

Methods:

1.   Patient Preparation. After the patient is moved to the operating room and anesthetized, the needle electrodes are placed by the surgeon in the forehead and in each earlobe and secured with surgical tape. The otologic surgeon then places the transtympanic needle electrode and the ear insert/probe microphone/sound delivery tube assembly. The audiologist connects the sound delivery and probe microphone tubes and checks the impedances of the electrodes. The impedance between the transtympanic needle electrode and the surface needle electrodes should be stable and less than 100 kohm. Satisfactory recordings have been obtained with stable impedances exceeding 100 kohm.

2.   <u>Baseline Recordings</u>. Before the patient is draped and while the patient is not being manipulated, baseline recordings and measurements of the probe microphone output are made. Click responses are obtained to 88 dB nHL condensation and rarefaction clicks. A determination is made as to which polarity produces the best response. That polarity will be used throughout the procedure. Tone burst responses are obtained for a 1-kHz tone (5 ms rise-fall, 5 ms plateau) to obtain CM and SP baseline values. An ABR will be obtained to 88 dB nHL rarefaction clicks. For endolymphatic sac procedures, alternating polarity clicks are used. The electrode configuration, stimulus and recording parameters are given in the Appendix A.

3.   <u>Monitoring</u>. After the baseline recordings are made, monitoring is performed at various intervals, depending on the progress of the surgery. Recordings should not be made during drilling, cautery, suction, probing for VII nerve location, or use of debulking instruments such as lasers and ultrasound devices. These procedures introduce excessive noise into the recording. Monitoring should be performed more frequently during times when the nerve is at high risk. These times are identified by the surgeon, who communicates this information to the audiologist. It may be necessary for the surgeon to pause occasionally during the surgical procedure in order to obtain adequate recordings. When a significant change occurs in latency or amplitude in the evoked potential, the surgeon is informed. For neurosurgical procedures, monitoring is terminated when the dura is closed or when the response has deteriorated to the point where changes cannot be detected and remains absent for at least 30 minutes. The video monitor, connected to the microscope camera, is used to relate recordings to surgical events throughout the procedure.

4.   <u>Shutdown</u>. When monitoring is terminated, all cables attached to the patient are disconnected from the computer before the equipment is turned off. All needle electrodes and sound tubes are discarded. The data file should be backed up before the equipment is turned off. Materials that have been in contact with the floor or patient (e.g., video cable, electrode junction box, electrode impedance meter, probe microphone preamplifier box and microphone/cable assembly, earphones) should be cleaned with decontamination solution before leaving the operating room area. Probe microphone preamplifier box should be shut off. Needle electrodes placed in the skin are placed in a "sharps" container.

Report Format:
A report is prepared on the hospital Progress Notes form that summarizes the course of intraoperative evoked potentials and includes a statement of prognosis for hearing preservation or relief from hydropic symptoms. (See Appendix C.)

Billing
Bill electrocochleography (CPT 92584) or auditory evoked potentials (CPT 92585) in 15-minute units.

References:
Møller, A. (1988). *Evoked Potentials in Intraoperative Monitoring*. Baltimore: Williams & Wilkins.

Desmedt, J. E. (Ed.). (1989). *Neuromonitoring in Surgery*. Amsterdam: Elsevier.

Levine, R. A. (1990). Short-latency auditory evoked potentials: Intraoperative applications. *International Anesthesiology Clinics, 28*, 147-153.

Protocol 17 Appendix

A.   Setup Parameters
B.   Intraoperative Monitoring Worksheet
C.   Intraoperative Auditory Monitoring Report

SETUP PARAMETERS

Electrode Configuration:

	Channel 1 (ABR)	Channel 2 (ECOG)
Active	Forehead	Promontory
Reference	Ipsilateral Earlobe	Forehead
Ground	Contralateral Earlobe	Contralateral Earlobe

Recording Parameters:

	Channel 1	Channel 2		
Gain:	100000	50000	Window:	Click 10 ms
High Filter:	1500	1500*		Tone 20 ms
Low Filter:	100	100*		
Notch Filter:	out	out	Points:	256
Art. Reject	enabled	disabled		

* For an endolymphatic sac procedure,	High Filter	3000
	Low Filter	3

Stimulus Parameters:

Transducer:	Insert
Stimuli:	Click (condensation, rarefaction, or alternating) 13/s (38/s for ABR)
	1 KHz tone burst (5 ms rise-fall, 5 ms plateau) 38/s
# of Stimuli	500 (more if needed)

INTRAOPERATIVE MONITORING WORKSHEET

PAGE ___

NAME: _____   HOSP. ID _____

BIRTHDATE ____-____-____   DATE ____-____-____

			R		L	
	CH1	CH2	CH1	CH2	CH1	CH2
ELECTRODE MONTAGE: ACTIVE ___ ___	ELECTRODE IMPEDANCE ___	___	___	___		

ELECTRODE MONTAGE: ACTIVE ___ ___   ELECTRODE IMPEDANCE ___ ___ ___ ___
                    REFERENCE ___ ___   ___ ___ ___ ___
                    GROUND ___ ___   ___ ___ ___ ___

PROCEDURE _____   SURGEON _____

RECORD	STIM	LEVEL	STIM RATE	STIM AMPL	NO. OF SWEEPS	COMMENT
1						
2						
3						
4						
5						
6						
7						
8						
9						
10						
11						
12						
13						
14						
15						
16						
17						
18						
19						
20						
21						

EVENT	TIME
INCISION	___
START CRANIOTOMY	___
FINISH CRANIOTOMY	___
OPEN DURA	___
EXPOSE TUMOR	___
START DRILLING T-BONE	___
FINISH DRILLING T-BONE	___
START RESECTING TUMOR	___
FINISH RESECTING TUMOR	___
SECTION NERVE	___
BEGIN N. DECOMPRESS	___
FINISH N. DECOMPRESS	___
	___
	___
	___
	___
	___
	___
	___

INTRAOPERATIVE AUDITORY MONITORING REPORT

Hosp ID #
Patient Name

3/24/94

Transtympanic electrocochleography (ECOG) and Auditory Brainstem Response (ABR) testing were performed intraoperatively during surgery for removal of a left acoustic neuroma to monitor auditory function. A needle electrode was placed on the promontory by Dr. L. Reference and ground electrodes were placed on the forehead and right earlobe, respectively. Stimuli were 88 dB nHL rarefaction clicks presented at a rate of 27/sec. The stimulus waveform was monitored with a probe microphone placed in the left ear canal.

The initial ECOG recordings were characterized by an action potential (AP) of approximately 2 microvolts and a latency of 4.24 msec. (See Auditory Evoked Potentials, ECOG Record 4) These values are consistent with the conductive hearing loss the patient exhibited in the pre-operative audiogram. During the drilling of the temporal bone, the response amplitude decreased while the latency increased slightly. (ECOG Record 9) The amplitude continued to decrease throughout the drilling until the response amplitude was too small to identify reliably. (Records 10, 11, 16) The final three recordings were averaged together and may show a small action potential. (Record 24, 25, 26)

The baseline ABR recording (ABR Record 4) showed abnormally delayed latency of Waves III and V, consistent with conductive hearing loss. No response was seen for the ABR at the conclusion of the surgery (ABR Record 26).

Upon removal of the drapes, the left ear canal was inspected with an otoscope. It appeared that the middle ear was filled with blood. There was blood in the ear canal and on the earplug that houses the sound delivery tube. The intraoperative changes in the AP and the ABR may have been caused by fluid in the middle ear. As a result, the prognosis for post-operative hearing cannot be determined from these results.

Audiologist

Section IV Cochlear Implants

Cochlear Implant Evaluation-Postlingual Adult

Target Population:
Postlingually deaf adult patients with severe to profound bilateral hearing impairment that may be cochlear implant candidates.

Rationale:
The purpose of the cochlear implant evaluation is to: a) obtain information to help determine whether the patient is an appropriate candidate for cochlear implantation; b) obtain preoperative baseline information; and c) provide counselling regarding cochlear implants.

Equipment Required:
Otoscope
Clinical audiometer (pure tone, speech and sound field capabilities)
Aural acoustic immittance system
Audio cassette recorder
Model of cochlear implant system
Surgeon's Handbook describing surgery
VCR and captioned videotape about cochlear implants
Sign language interpreter if necessary (this must be arranged in advance)

Methods:
The complete evaluation will require an extended appointment because of the time needed to both counsel the patient and complete the testing. The evaluation includes a) Basic Hearing Evaluation (Protocol 1); b) evaluation of the patient's amplification; c) speech recognition evaluation; d) evaluation of lipreading enhancement; e) consultation to explain the implant system and the process of getting a cochlear implant; and, f) administration and discussion of expectations questionnaires.

1.   History. Obtain a detailed history of the hearing problem. Information about the patient's past and current mode(s) of communication using the Cochlear Implant Patient Information form (Appendix A) is obtained on the phone prior to the evaluation. Requests are made for previous audiologic data.

2.   Basic Hearing Evaluation. A basic hearing evaluation as described in Protocol 1 including multifrequency tympanometry, will be completed. Word recognition testing with NU-6 materials under phones is presented if the signal can be made sufficiently audible to the patient. Otherwise, speech recognition testing will be done with the patient's amplification as in Step 5. If pseudohypacusis is suspected, Auditory Brainstem Response testing (Protocol 14) should be conducted. If the patient does not respond to pure tones under headphones at any

frequency, a promontory stimulation test should be scheduled for a subsequent visit (see Step 10).

3.   <u>Hearing Aid Electroacoustic Measures</u>. If the patient has hearing aids, an Electroacoustic Hearing Aid Evaluation (Protocol 12) should be conducted to determine if the aids are functioning properly.

4.   <u>Hearing Aid Sound Field Measures</u>. Functional gain should be measured in the sound field with the patient's amplification as described in Protocol 8. This method is used rather than real-ear measurements since it is impossible to use real-ear measures with cochlear implants and functional gain provides at least a gross means of comparison between use of the hearing aid and use of the cochlear implant.

5.   <u>Speech Recognition Testing</u>. This testing is performed in the patient's best-aided condition in the sound field using the tape recorded cochlear implant speech recognition test battery. The tests should be presented at 50 dB HL or at a higher level if necessary to make the stimuli audible to the patient. The patient is given the test sheet and the audiologist reviews the written instructions to make sure the patient understands the task. The audiologist should encourage guessing and observe the patient during testing to make sure the patient performs the task appropriately. The test battery includes a 4-choice spondee test, CID Everyday Sentence Test, NU-6 Monosyllable Word Test (50 word list), Iowa Vowel Recognition, and Medial Consonant Recognition tests. Occasionally, Iowa Sentences Without Context Test are included to confirm the CID sentence results.

Begin with the 4-choice spondee test. This is the easiest test and though it is not diagnostically significant, it serves to acquaint the patient with the testing format. Next, complete the CID Everyday Sentence Test and the NU-6 Monosyllable Word Test.

If the patient scores $\geq$ 45% on CID sentences and $\geq$ 28% on NU-6 words, the patient is not a cochlear implant candidate. See Step 7, Criteria for Candidacy.

If the patient scores < 45% on CID sentences and < 28% on NU-6 words, complete the remainder of the speech recognition battery including the lipreading enhancement tests (Step 6).

6.   <u>Lipreading Enhancement</u>. This test uses CID sentences and is presented live-voice by the audiologist, who is seated in front of the patient. The test is first performed without amplification in a lipreading only condition. The audiologist reads the list of sentences and the patient responds by repeating as much of the sentence as able. The test is then repeated with a different list of CID sentences and the patient uses amplification and lipreading. The amount of lipreading enhancement is the difference between the lipreading only and the lipreading plus sound scores. This measure gives an indication of the patient's communicative ability in everyday situations.

7.   <u>Criteria for Candidacy</u>. If the patient scores < 35% on the CID Everyday Sentence Test and < 10% on the NU 6 Monosyllabic Word Test, the patient is not receiving significant speech understanding benefit from amplification, and meets the audiologic criteria for cochlear implant candidacy. Proceed to Step 8: Counseling.

If the patient scores $\geq$ 45% on the CID Everyday Sentence Test and $\geq$ 28% on the NU-6

Monosyllabic Word Test, the patient is receiving too much hearing aid benefit to be considered a cochlear implant candidate. The patient should be counseled regarding this and encouraged to return should changes occur.

Scores between 35% and 45% on CID sentences or 10 - 28% on NU-6 represent a "gray area" and other factors may need to be considered such as a difference between ears, the patient's age, length of deafness, and the amount of lipreading enhancement the patient receives with amplification. If these patients receive greater than 85% on the hearing aid plus lipreading subtest, they are performing as well as or better than the average cochlear implant patient and they should be counseled that they are not a candidate at this time because the implant may not be able to improve their present level of communication functioning. If they score less than 85% in the combined condition, they still may be a candidate. See Appendix F for FDA recommended Patient Selection Criteria.

8.   Counseling. If the patient appears to be a candidate, he/she is to be thoroughly counseled about all aspects of the cochlear implant and the process for obtaining it. Using the Cochlear Implant Counseling Checklist (Appendix D) as a guide, the following information should be given to the patient:

   a.   Explain ear anatomy, normal hearing and sensorineural hearing loss using a model or illustration of the ear.

   b.   Explain the concept of how a cochlear implant electrically stimulates the hearing nerve to provide "hearing" sensation.

   c.   Show the patient the internal receiver/stimulator unit and the electrode array. Use the illustrations in the Surgeon's Handbook to show how the device is implanted.

   d.   Show the patient the speech processor and microphone headset. Use the illustrations to show the relationship between the internal and external components of the implant system. Explain the pathway taken by the incoming sound as it is processed and sent to the electrode array.

   e.   Explain the expected benefits of the cochlear implant:

   Sound Quality. Most patients receive a restored sensation of sound including an awareness of environmental sounds and speech. Emphasize that the implant does not provide normal hearing. Most patients describe the sound quality as unnatural and/or mechanical.

   Speech Recognition. Most patients find that they can understand speech best when using lipreading in combination with sound from the implant. Some patients cannot understand speech at all with the implant unless they are lipreading at the same time. A few patients can understand open-set speech with the implant alone and without visual cues.

   Telephone Use. Telephone abilities vary greatly from patient to patient. Some cannot use the phone at all, others only with familiar voices and a few are able to carry on lengthy phone conversations. Emphasize that it is impossible to predict before the operation whether or not a person will be able to use the phone.

   Environmental Sounds. Environmental sounds will often sound different than the patient remembers and may need to be relearned.

   Music. Because the speech processor is designed to process speech, it is not likely that music enjoyment will return.

   Implant versus Hearing Aid. The implant sounds very different from a hearing aid. In some cases a cochlear implant is not as natural, but it may provide better speech understanding than a hearing aid for appropriate candidates.

Training. Because the sound is different from normal hearing, it is necessary to undergo training to learn how to use the new sound. Give the patient a copy of Cochlear Implant Expectations (Appendix E).

f.   Explain that the surgery is performed while the patient is under general anesthesia and takes approximately 3 hours. The patient checks into the hospital at 5:30 am on the morning of surgery and usually remains in the hospital for one or two nights. Patients return to the clinic in about 10 days to have their incision site checked for proper healing. It is necessary to allow the surgical site to heal for about 4-5 weeks before the patient returns for the external parts of the implant system.

g.   Show the cochlear implant video if appropriate. (If the patient is prelingually deaf the tape is inappropriate because prelingually deafened adults receive less benefit than the postlingual patients shown on the tape.)

h.   Explain the remaining evaluation to determine candidacy i.e. CT scans to make sure the cochlea is patent, psychological questionnaires and interview, expectations questionnaires, promontory stimulation to determine if the hearing nerve can respond to the implant, balance testing, and a consultation with the surgeon.

i.   Describe the hook-up, programming, rehabilitation and follow-up testing. The initial hook-up includes three visits the first week, (with the first two on consecutive days), one visit the 2nd, 4th, and 7th week, with the interval dependant on the patients needs and problems. Follow-up testing consists of repeating the speech recognition battery at 3 months, 6 months, 12 months and then yearly.

j.   Discuss the costs of getting an implant, including the initial evaluation, the surgery, the device, and programming during the first year. If the insurance company does not list the clinic as a provider, it will be necessary to obtain a referral from the primary care physician for each visit to ensure reimbursement. Most insurance companies require prior authorization for cochlear implant surgery.

k.   Answer any questions the patient and family may have.

9.   Expectations Questionnaires. These are true-false questionnaires that are given to the patient and also to any friends or family members who may be present. The audiologist reviews the answers and discusses them, attempting to correct any false notions about the cochlear implant.

10.   Psychological Questionnaires. Implant candidates are also asked to fill out the Beck Inventory, the Spielberger Self-Evaluation Questionnaire, and the Personal Expectations Questionnaire just prior to the Psychology evaluation. These will be reviewed by the Health Psychologist. In addition, the patient should complete the Profile for Profound and Severe Hearing Loss.

11.   Promontory Stimulation Test. This test is used to determine whether a cochlear implant candidate can experience auditory sensations from electrical stimulation of the cochlea. It is done if no response is obtained to pure tones under headphones. It is conducted in the otolaryngology clinic and involves the cochlear implant surgeon, a nurse and the audiologist. The eardrum is anesthetized by the nurse and the surgeon inserts a needle electrode transtympanically through the eardrum and places it on the promontory. The audiologist delivers electrical pulses to the cochlea and looks for the patient's behavioral response (raising of the hand or tapping of the finger) indicating an electrical threshold has been obtained. Patients who do not exhibit a consistent "auditory" response (vibrotactile response is not sufficient) to electrical stimulation of the promontory are not considered candidates for implantation.

Report   Format:
Results will be recorded on the Audiologic Record Form (Appendix G) and on the Patient Speech Recognition Profile Form (Appendix C). A narrative report will be included in the patient's hospital chart and appropriate reports will be sent to referral sources.

Billing:
For the first visit the patient will be billed for a Basic Hearing Evaluation as according to Protocol1. Promontory stimulation testing should be billed as one unit of Promontory Stimulation (CPT 92599) for each 15-minute unit spent with the patient.

References:

Cochlear Implants in Adults and Children. National Institute of Health Consensus Development Conference Statement, May 1995, 15-17.

Filsch, K. S., Fisher, S. G., Westen, S. C., & Shapiro, W. H. (1992). Evaluation and adaptation of a cochlear implant test battery. *Seminars in Hearing, 13*, 208-217.

Gantz, B. J., Abbas, P. J., Knutson, J. F., Tyler, R. S., & Woodworth, G. G. (1993). Multivariate predictors of audiological success with multichannel cochlear implants. *Annals of Otology, Rhinology & Laryngology, 102*, 909-916.

Kimberley, B. P., Lee, A. M., Scheller, L. D., Levine, S. C., Adams, G. L., & Nelson, D. A. (1989).   Cochlear implant hearing performance at the University of Minnesota. *Journal of Otolaryngology, 18*, 24-27.

Pope, M. C. (1991). Readiness issues in candidate selection. *American Journal of Otology, 12* Supplement, 81.

Skinner, M. W., Clark, G. M., Whitford, L. A., Seligman, P. M., Staller, S. J., Shipp, D. B., Shallop, J. K., Everingham, C., Menapace, C. M., Arndt, P. L., Antogenelli, T., Brimacombe, J. A., Pijl, S., Daniels, P., George, C. R., McDermott, H. J., & Beiter, A. L. (1994). Evaluation of a new spectral peak coding strategy for the Nucleus 22 channel cochlear implant system. *The American Journal of Otology, 15*, 15-27.

Tyler, R. S., & Kelsey, D. (1990). Advantages and disadvantages reported by some of the better cochlear implant patients. *American Journal of Otology, 11*, 282-289.

Wilson, B. S., Lawson, D. T., Finley, C. C., & Wolford, R. D. (1993). Importance of patient and processor variables in determining outcomes with cochlear implants. *Journal of Speech and Hearing Research, 36*, 373-379.

Yune, H. Y., Miyamoto, R. T., & Yune, M. E. (1991). Medical imaging in cochlear implant candidates. *American Journal of Otology, 12*, 11-17.

Protocol 18 Appendix

A.   Cochlear Implant Patient Information
B.   Cochlear Implant Pre-Operative Evaluation Checklist--Postlingual Adults
C.   Patient Speech Recognition Profile
D.   Cochlear Implant Counseling Checklist
E.   Cochlear Implant Expectations
F.   Postlingual Adult Patient Selection Criteria for Cochlear Implant

COCHLEAR IMPLANT PATIENT INFORMATION

Date:

Name:

Address: _

Phone: _   (home)
                                 (work)

DOB: _   Age: UH#:

Contact Person:

Referred By:

INSURANCE INFORMATION:

<u>Primary Insurer</u>   <u>Supplemental Insurance</u>

Company: _

Address:

Insured: _

ID#: _

Group#:

Other:

PATIENT HISTORY:

When was hearing loss first noticed? _

Etiology? _

Has patient ever had ear surgery?

Age of onset of profound hearing loss:

# of years of profound hearing loss: Age of initial amplification:

COCHLEAR IMPLANT PATIENT INFORMATION *page 2*

Current amplification?

Length of time patient has had present amplification: _

Length of time since amplification last worn: _

Telephone use with hearing aid? _

Current mode of communication:

Lipreading ability?

Intelligibility of patient's speech:

Any medical problems with might contraindicate surgery?

Education:

Employment:

Where did the patient hear about cochlear implants?

ADDITIONAL INFORMATION:

Cochlear Implant Pre-Operative Evaluation Checklist--Postlingual Adults

Initial Consultation

Air and Bone Conduction Thresholds

Tympanometry and Acoustic Reflexes

Electroacoustic evaluation of hearing aids

Functional Gain in Sound Field

ABR   (optional)

Psychological Questionnaires

Psychological Interview

Vision Test (optional)

ENG

CT scans of the temporal bones

Promontory Stimulation

SPEECH RECOGNITION TESTING

4-Choice Spondee

Vowel Recognition

Medial Consonant

Monosyllabic Words (NU6)

CID Sentences

Iowa Sentences

LIPREADING ENHANCEMENT MEASURES
(CID Sentences)

Lipreading Only

Lipreading + Sound

Expectations Questionnaire

PATIENT SPEECH RECOGNITION PROFILE

Name: Audiologist:

Closed-Set Subtests

	Pre	3 Mo.	6 Mo.	1 Yr.	2 Yr.	3 Yr.	4 Yr.	5 Yr.
4-Choice Spondee								
Vowel								
Medial Consonant								
Presentation Level in dB HL								

Open-Set Subtests

	Pre	3 Mo.	6 Mo.	1 Yr.	2 Yr.	3 Yr.	4 Yr	5 Yr.
CID Sentences								
NU#6								
Iowa Sentences								
Presentation Level in dB HL								

Lipreading Enhancement

	Pre	3 Mo.	6 Mo.	1 Yr.	2 Yr.	3 Yr.	4 Yr	5 Yr.
Lipreading only								
Lipreading & Sound								
Lipreading & Implant & Sound								

COCHLEAR IMPLANT COUNSELING CHECKLIST

Explain sensorineural hearing loss using an illustration of the ear.

Explain the concept of using an implant to provide electrical hearing.

Explain the model of the internal implant.

Explain the speech processor and microphone headset.

Explain the expected benefits of the implant:

> sound awareness,
> does not provide normal hearing,
> sound quality,
> speech recognition,
> telephone use,
> environmental sounds,
> music,
> difference between implant and hearing aid,
> training

Explain the surgery and hospital stay.

Show the implant video if appropriate.

Explain the remaining evaluation to determine candidacy.

Explain the hook-up, rehabilitation and follow-up testing.

Explain the costs and the process of getting insurance authorization.

COCHLEAR IMPLANT EXPECTATIONS

ENVIRONMENTAL SOUNDS----

will sound different than you remember them. It is necessary to relearn many environmental sounds as many of them may sound similar to each other. For some implant users, the environmental sounds seem more like they remember after some training and time to become accustomed to listening with the implant. For others, the environmental sounds may always sound different than before the hearing loss. If you had been using a hearing aid prior to receiving the implant, the sounds will probably be much different with the implant, less "natural" than with the hearing aid.

MUSIC----

does not sound pleasant to most implant users. Many report that it sounds like static or like noise. It may be possible to enjoy a single instrument, such as a clarinet playing a simple tune or a single voice singing, but a big orchestra or a complex piece with many instruments playing at once will probably just sound jumbled and noisy. Part of the reason for this is because the Nucleus implant is designed to code information for speech and this is different than the information needed for music. A few implant users do enjoy music, but don't count on it!

BACKGROUND NOISES----

may always be a problem because they can interfere with trying to listen to speech. Normal hearing people have a problem with this too but they are able to "tune out" the noise to focus on what they want to listen to. When people lose their hearing they also lose their ability to listen selectively. If you are using your implant in a noisy place you may be able to improve the situation by using "S", the noise suppression setting. Many people notice that while the "S" setting decreases the volume of the background noise, it also decreases the volume of the speech. Another solution is to try using the handheld microphone that plugs into the processor to improve the signal to noise ratio.

SPEECH----

Lipreading will always be a major part of your communication even with the implant. Most patients find that is works best this way. The implant can help make it easier to separate one word from the next in normal conversation. It will be possible to hear your own voice so you can regulate the volume of your own speech. You may be able to tell the difference between voices of people that you know well. It should be fairly easy to tell the difference between male and female voices. Speech will not sound the same as you remember it, especially not at first. It is necessary to undergo a period of training and adjustment of the processor to learn to recognize the new speech sounds. Speech may even sound annoying for the first few days until you get used to the processor and we determine the best program for your device. With time, voices may seem to sound almost normal to you but this is not true for everyone. Some patients will be able to recognize various amounts of speech without lipreading and may be able to make some use of the telephone but there is no way to predict beforehand whether or not you would be able to do this. Your hearing will never be normal with the implant and will not become normal after you wear the device for a long time. Everyone who has the implant does not develop the same hearing abilities. Some patients do better than others and we are not sure at the present time why this occurs. Unfortunately, we have no way to predict the success of a given

COCHLEAR IMPLANT EXPECTATIONS *page 2*

individual. The majority of patients who receive the implant feel that it is a tremendous help to them and significantly improves their ability to communicate. Most still have communication problems in some situations, however.

THE FIRST FEW DAYS----

after your hook-up may or may not be exciting ones. Most new users complain that the sound is very high-pitched and unnatural. Part of the reason it seems high-pitched is because it is. The electrodes lie in the basal or high frequency end of the cochlea.

Fortunately, the brain has a marvelous ability to adjust to new stimulation and most people report that the sound seems more natural to them after they have worn it for a few weeks. For a few people, the processor seems to always sound high-pitched. Sometimes we can adjust the processor or eliminate some of the highest pitched electrodes in the program, but this is not always successful. Almost every patient reports that the sound of the implant improves over time even though you may find this difficult to believe as you listen to it on the first day! Consistent use (12 or more hours a day) is important for adjusting to the implant system.

IF YOU HAVE BEEN WEARING A HEARING AID----

sounds will be different with the implant. For most patients, the implant will give more help in understanding speech than the hearing aid and many patients discontinue wearing their hearing aid after receiving the implant. Some patients find that they like the quality of the environmental sounds better with their hearing aid and they may choose to wear the hearing aid on the side opposite the implant. Even though the sounds are very different, some people seem to be able to integrate the implant signal and the sounds from the hearing aid quite well. The hearing aid can help "fill-in" those low frequency sounds that the implant may miss while conversely, the implant provides the high frequencies missed by the hearing aid.

POSTLINGUAL ADULT PATIENT SELECTION CRITERIA FOR COCHLEAR IMPLANT

1.   Severe to profound sensorineural hearing loss bilaterally with a postlingual onset (usually defined as after age 5)

2.   18 years of age or older

3.   Little or no benefit from hearing aids (as defined by poor performance on open-set tests of speech recognition,i.e., 30% or less on CID sentences and Iowa sentences)

4.   No radiological contraindications to placing the electrodes or receiver (CT scans must be reviewed by the surgeon)

5.   No medical contraindications for surgery or rehabilitation

6.   Positive response to promontory stimulation

7.   Psychologically and motivationally suitable

Protocol 19 Cochlear Implant Evaluation-Child

Target Population:
Children aged 2-17 who are being considered for a multi-channel cochlear implant.

Rationale:
The purpose is to: a) obtain information to help determine whether the child is an appropriate candidate for a cochlear implant; b) obtain baseline information; and c) educate the parents and child about the cochlear implant system.

Equipment Required:
Otoscope
Clinical audiometer (puretone, speech and soundfield capability)
Variety of toys for conditioned play audiometry
Aural acoustic immittance system
Audio cassette recorder
Electroacoustic hearing aid measurement system
Model of cochlear implant system
Surgeon's handbook describing surgery
VCR and captioned videotape about cochlear implants
Sign language interpreter as appropriate

Methods:
Optimally, the evaluation should take two visits. The first would include the pediatric hearing evaluation (Protocol 4), aided threshold for soundfield warble tones, and counseling. Before the second visit, the child should have an ENT examination, and a CT scan. A psychological and speech and language assessment will be obtained. These can be completed externally or at this clinic. The second visit would include speech recognition evaluation, measurement of speechreading with and without sound, and conclude with a discussion of cochlear implant candidacy.

1.   History. Parents are required to send in the Pediatric History Questionnaire, the Family Questionnaire and pertinent medical, audiological and school information about the child prior to scheduling the evaluation. (See Appendix A-E.) This information should be reviewed by the audiologists before the child is seen.

2.   Basic Hearing Evaluation. Depending on the age and capabilities of the child, obtain pure tone threshold information as described in Protocol 1, Basic Hearing Evaluation. Younger children may require Conditioned Play Audiometry as described in Protocol 4, Pediatric Hearing Evaluation. (Note that for deaf children, it is important to begin conditioning with vibrotactile stimulation through the bone conduction vibrator.) Acoustic immittance measures should be completed as indicated in Protocol 1, Basic Hearing Evaluation.

3.   Aided Thresholds for Soundfield Warble Tones. Evaluate the child's amplification by performing an Electroacoustic Hearing Aid Evaluation as in Protocol 12. Check to see that the child's earmolds fit properly and that the hearing aids can be turned up to an adequate output level before feedback. Obtain aided soundfield thresholds for warble tones (See Protocol 8, Hearing Aid Fitting, Method 2b).

4.   Speech Recognition Evaluation. Using appropriate amplification, the following tests may be used to assess the child's speech recognition ability depending on the child's age and abilities:

Closed set	Open set
CID Early Speech Perception Battery (standard or low-verbal version)	GASP Words and Sentences
	Common Phrase Test
NU-CHIPS	CID Sentences
Minimal Pairs Test	PBK Words
	MI Potato Head Test

5.   Measurement of Speechreading With and Without Sound. Use either the Craig Lipreading Test for young children or the CID Sentences for older children with well-developed English language skills.

6.   Counseling. Explaining the cochlear implant system, appropriate expectations, and the process of obtaining an implant to the parents. Follow the Parent Counseling Checklist in Appendix F and the Pediatric Patient Selection Criteria in Appendix G. It is important that older children and teenagers take part in the decision to implant since the success of the implant depends on their willing cooperation in learning to use and wear the device. If the child is over age 10 (or if the parents feel a younger child should be included) have a sign language interpreter present to help explain the implant to the child. Older children should take part in the discussion. Care must be taken to ensure that they want the device for themselves and not just to please parents and teachers. If the child has not had an adequate trial with amplification, this should be recommended for an appropriate period (usually at least six months) and the child should be reevaluated after the trial period. Emphasis should be placed on the commitment necessary for successful cochlear implant use.

7.   Other Considerations. Final determination of a child's candidacy can only be made after the child undergoes CT scans, a psychological evaluation and a speech/language baseline evaluation. (See Appendix G for Pediatric Patient Selection Criteria and Contraindications.)

Report Format:
Audiometric results will be recorded on the Audiologic Record Form. Results of speech-recognition and lipreading measures will be recorded on the forms for each test and will be described in the Audiology report. (See Appendix H.) This information should be directed to the child's physician, school, rehabilitation personnel (if applicable), and parents.

Billing:

Bill for standard audiometric procedures as in Protocol 4, Pediatric Hearing Evaluation.

References:

Advanced Bionics Corporation. (1995).   *Clarion™ Multi-Strategy Cochlear Implant Pediatric Clinical Investigation.*

Cochlear Corporation. (1990).   *Nucleus® 22-Channel Cochlear Implant System: Pediatric Procedures Manual.*

Geers, A. (1994).   Techniques for assessing auditory speech perception and lipreading enhancement in young deaf children. *The Volta Review, 96,* 85-96.

Mecklenburg, D. J. (1988).   Cochlear implants in children: Nonmedical considerations. *American Journal of Otology, 9,* 163-168.

Northern, J. L., Black, O. F., Brimacombe, J. A., Cohen, N. L., Eisenberg, L. S., Kuprenas, S. V., Martinez, S. A., & Mischke, R. E. (1986).   Selection of children for cochlear implantation. *Seminars in Hearing, 7,* 341-347.

Roeser, R. J., & Yellin, W. (1987).   Pure-tone tests with preschool children.   In F. N. Martin (Ed.), *Hearing Disorders in Children* (pp. 217-264). Austin: Pro-Ed.

Staller, S. J., Beiter, A. L., & Brimacombe, J. A. (1994).   Use of the Nucleus 22 Channel cochlear implant system with children. *The Volta Review, 96,* 15-39.

Tyler, R. S. (1993)   *Cochlear Implants: Audiological Foundations.* San Diego: Singular Publishing Group, Inc.

Protocol 19 Appendix

A.   University of Minnesota Children's Cochlear Implant Program
B.   Pediatric History
C.   Family Questionnaire
D.   School Information Release
E.   Health Insurance Information
F.   Parent Counseling Checklist
G.   Pediatric Patient Selection Criteria
H.   Example of Pediatric Cochlear Implant Report

UNIVERSITY OF MINNESOTA CHILDREN'S COCHLEAR IMPLANT PROGRAM

Please send the following information about your child. It is important that we receive this information <u>before</u> we can schedule an initial visit for your child:

Pediatric History and Family Questionnaire. Please fill these out and return them to the Cochlear Implant Program.

Medical Recordspertaining to the hearing loss and any associated health or developmental problems. Sign the enclosed <u>Patient Information Release</u> form and send it to your child's doctor and they will forward the information to us.

School Records. Please sign the enclosed <u>School Information Release</u> form and return it to the Cochlear Implant Program in the enclosed envelope. This gives us permission to receive your child's school records and communicate with his/her teachers. We will send the Release to the school along with a packet of information about the cochlear implant to inform the school that your child is being evaluated and enlist their help in the process.

Health Insurance Information. Please fill out the enclosed <u>Health Insurance Information</u> form an return it to the Cochlear Implant Program. We will begin the prior authorization process by sending out a letter to your insurance company describing the implant and asking if they will cover the costs. (It often takes a couple of months to receive a reply from the insurance company so we prefer to start this process as soon as possible.)

PEDIATRIC HISTORY

DATE

CHILD'S NAME	AGE	GRADE

PARENT'S NAME(S)

WHO REFERRED YOU TO US?

DESCRIBE YOUR CHILD'S PROBLEM:

DO YOU HAVE CONCERNS ABOUT HOW YOUR CHILD HEARS?
DESCRIBE:
    DOES YOUR CHILD:
        a. Respond if you call him/her from another room?   ❏ Yes ❏ No
        b. Respond to his/her name?   ❏ Yes ❏ No
        c. Try to look toward the sound source when a noise is made? ❏ Yes ❏ No
        d. Alert to familiar sounds - for example a spoon in a cup? ❏ Yes ❏ No
        e. Stop what he/she is doing when there is an unfamiliar sound? ❏ Yes ❏ No

DO YOU HAVE ANY CONCERNS ABOUT HOW YOUR CHILD TALKS?
DESCRIBE:
    DOES YOUR CHILD:
        a. Say at least 10 words?   ❏ Yes ❏ No
        b. Say 2-3 word sentences?   ❏ Yes ❏ No
        c. Speak clearly to the family?   ❏ Yes ❏ No

NAME OF CHILD'S SCHOOL:

DO YOU HAVE CONCERNS ABOUT YOUR CHILD'S BEHAVIOR (TANTRUMS, HITTING, WILL NOT
FOLLOW DIRECTIONS, ETC.) AT SCHOOL, HOME OR IN THE NEIGHBORHOOD?
DESCRIBE:

IS YOUR CHILD HAVING ANY PROBLEMS LEARNING AT SCHOOL?
DESCRIBE:

DO YOU NOTE ANY PROBLEMS WITH YOUR CHILD'S GENERAL DEVELOPMENT?
DESCRIBE:

  AT APPROXIMATELY WHAT AGE DID YOUR CHILD:
        a. Roll over   c. Crawl   e. Say his/her first word
        b. Sit up   d. Walk   f. Toilet train

ARE THERE ANY PROBLEMS WITH YOUR CHILD'S GENERAL HEALTH (PLEASE INCLUDE EAR
INFECTION HISTORY)?
DESCRIBE:

FAMILY QUESTIONNAIRE

Child's Name: **Age:**   **Date:**

General Behavior

Does child fall frequently?   How well can s/he climb?   Throw a ball?

Ride a two-wheel bike?   Run?   _ Which hand is used for eating and/or drawing with?

What time does s/he go to bed?   Get up?   Does the child take a nap?

If so, at what time?   _ How well does the child play alone?   With other children?

Does the child enjoy books?   Does s/he like to watch TV?   For how long?

Describe the   child's free-time activities

Describe the child's friends

Below is a list of words that describe children's personality and behavior. Please circle those that describe your child.

sad	leader	follower	has temper tantrums
quiet	happy	affectionate	has trouble sleeping
dependent	independent	moody	prefers to be alone
even tempered	very active	sucks thumb	is usually fearful
happy	friendly		

Describe any behavior that is a problem

Does your child receive help in: Feeding?   Toileting?   Dressing?   Bathing?

What age do you think your child is most like in regard to:
     Using his/her body and hands   Making sounds or talking

     Understanding what you say   Thinking and solving problems

     Playing with toys or other children

Does your child have unusual fears: If yes, please explain.

From which family activities has this child been excluded?

What do you consider to be your child's strengths?

In what ways do you treat this child differently from your other child/children?

Has the child ever failed to progress or lost any previously achieved skills? If yes, please explain.

FAMILY QUESTIONNAIRE *page 2*

Communication Status
Previous audiological findings: Degree of loss

Does the child wear a hearing aid?   Right ear   Left ear   Model/Type

How old was your child when s/he first obtained aid(s)?

How many hours a day does the child wear the aid(s)?

Does the child seem to enjoy wearing the aid?

What method of communication is used at home and at school?

> Oral/auditory (listening, lipreading, speaking)
> Total communication (sign language plus speech)
> Sign language only/ ASL

Has your child previously received or is presently receiving special therapy (speech and language, auditory training, or other)? If yes, please describe.

Educational Setting
Describe the child's educational setting (home programming, classroom with deaf and hard-of-hearing, regular classroom with a sign language interpreter, etc.)

How do you feel the child is progressing in this setting?

Name and address of school child currently attends:

Please give the names(s) of the child's primary teachers and phone numbers (include special education teachers and other rehabilitation services)

SCHOOL INFORMATION RELEASE

Student's Name   Birthdate

School Name

School Address

Name of Child's Primary Teacher

My child is being considered for a cochlear implant at the University of Minnesota. Before an evaluation can be scheduled, the following school records should be sent to the University:

> Most recent audiogram

> Most recent speech and language assessment

> Current IEP

> Reports from any other special services, i.e. physical therapy, psychology, etc.

> Any other pertinent information which may be useful in determining candidacy and future rehabilitation

> Please send to:

Parent Signature   Date

HEALTH INSURANCE INFORMATION

Patient name:

Policy holder's name:

ID#:   Group#

Other:

Insurance Company Name:

Address:

Phone:

If the patient is covered under more than one type of insurance, please list the primary insurance company above and give the same information for the supplemental insurance in the space below.

PARENT COUNSELING CHECKLIST

How the ear hears sounds. Hearing-impaired ears.

How the cochlear implant works. Electrical stimulation of the hearing nerve. Implant system consists of the internal device, the speech processor and the microphone headset. Implant system pathway to deliver sound to the inner ear.

Implant benefits with adults. Sound awareness, speech recognition with and without lipreading. Differences between postlingual and prelingual adults.

Expected implant benefits with children. Results with Nucleus device. Time lag between getting device and seeing improvement.

> Restored sound sensation

> Sound quality differences

> Understanding speech

Evaluation to determine candidacy. Audiological, medical, speech-language, psychology, family commitment, educational.

Surgery and Hospital stay.

Hook-up, and Device Setting.

Rehabilitation. Will take place in the school setting.

Follow-up Testing. 6 month intervals after initial hook-up completed.

Cost. Insurance prior authorization.

Deaf Culture

PEDIATRIC PATIENT SELECTION CRITERIA AND CONTRAINDICATIONS

1.   Patients should demonstrate a profound-to-total, bilateral sensorineural hearing loss.

2.   Ages 2-17

3.   Patients should demonstrate little or no benefit from a hearing aid as defined by obtaining virtually zero on open-set speech recognition measures and/or chance performance on closed-set segmental tasks.

3.   Radiological contraindications for placement of the receiver-stimulator or the electrode should not be present.

4.   Medical contraindications for undergoing implant surgery and rehabilitation should not be present.

5.   Families and (if possible) candidates should be well-motivated and possess appropriate expectations.

6.   Candidates, families and educational facilities should be prepared and willing to participate in and cooperate with pre- and postoperative training and assessment programs.

7.   Candidates should be enrolled in educational settings that emphasize oral/aural training.

8.   Normal intelligence and without additional handicaps that would have a negative impact on implant use.

9.   Candidates should have received at least six months of consistent exposure to input from a sensory aid (e.g., hearing aid, vibrotactile device, or cochlear implant). If a child has not had an appropriate trial with amplification, this should be recommended both to ensure that the child's ability to use a sensory device is assessed fairly and to ensure that the parents and educators are willing to follow through with recommendations.

10.   Adolescents should demonstrate spontaneous, differentiated vocalizations during communication.

Contraindications

1.   Medical contraindications to surgery.

2.   Deafness due to lesions of the acoustic nerve or central auditory pathway.

3.   Active acute middle ear infections.

4.   Presence of cochlear ossification that prevents electrode insertion may be a contraindication depending upon the extent of the ossification.

5.   Presence of problems related to limited skull maturation (e.g., Treacher Collins, etc.)

PEDIATRIC PATIENT SELECTION CRITERIA AND CONTRAINDICATIONS *page 2*

6. Absence of cochlear or eighth nerve development.

7. Significant benefit from acoustic amplification.

8. Congenital anomalies of the facial nerve.

EXAMPLE OF AN AUDIOLOGIC REPORT

December 5, 1995

Re:
UH#:
DOB
DOE

AUDIOLOGIC REPORT

HISTORY: Jennifer was seen at this clinic for a cochlear implant evaluation. She has a previously reported profound hearing impairment which was suspected to be present since shortly after birth. However, the exact etiology is unknown. Jennifer was premature and in a Neonatal Intensive Care Unit. She was initially diagnosed at about one year of age. Auditory brainstem response testing completed locally showed no responses to click stimuli presented to each ear. Behavioral testing showed minimal responses with hearing aid use. She is wearing binaural Phonak Pico Forte PP-C-L 2 behind-the-ear hearing aids for the last two years. However, her mother indicated that over the last several months, she has had intermittent hearing aid use.

Jennifer is attending a program for the deaf and hard of hearing, where they are utilizing total communication. Jennifer has a sign vocabulary of 60 words and is not verbalizing. She has balance problems for which she is receiving physical therapy. Communication with her educators suggest their support for cochlear implant use, but they have some apprehension about the amount of benefit potential.

EXAMINATION: Present testing utilized play audiometric procedures. Jennifer readily conditioned to bone conduction stimuli. However, with auditory input, she only responded to 250 Hz in the left ear at 100 dB HL unaided. It is assumed that she understood the task as when vibrotactile stimuli and the 250 Hz intense signal were presented, Jennifer consistently responded to the task. Tympanograms for both ears were normally shaped, which suggests normal tympanic membrane mobility. Acoustic reflexes were absent, consistent with her degree of hearing impairment.

An electroacoustic assessment of her hearing aids showed them to be in good working order and meeting manufacturer's specifications. With these instruments in place she only responded to a 250-Hz warble tone at 70 dB HL. The Early Speech Perception test was attempted but she was not able to do any discriminations, with auditory or visual and lipreading cues.

CONSULTATION: Extensive information was provided on the cochlear implant device, how it functions within the auditory system, some of the expected performance with cochlear implant use, which included the large range of benefits received with different age levels, and different children. Also included were the risks of surgery and possible problems with the device itself. Finally, Jennifer's parents were informed of the political climate within the deaf culture community relative to cochlear implant use. They were encouraged to talk to deaf adults before making their final decision. The necessity of auxiliary rehabilitation was emphasized as the classroom setting indicated that they do not have the resources to provide all the needed individual therapy.

EXAMPLE OF AN AUDIOLOGIC REPORT *page 2*

OTOLOGIC: A CT scan was completed prior to their visit with Dr._____ . On reviewing the scans, there were no medical contraindications to cochlear implant use. Information about the surgical procedure and the risks of the surgery were presented.

PSYCHOLOGIC: Psychologic evaluation was completed by Dr._____ . A summary of this evaluation suggested that Jennifer, although showing significant speech and language delays, performance ability for non language tests and scales at age appropriate levels.

SUMMARY AND RECOMMENDATIONS: Findings reflect a profound bilateral hearing impairment for which Jennifer is deriving only minimal benefit from her personal amplification. In consideration of the assessments at this facility and input from her educations, a cochlear implant is being recommended. The specified ear is the left as this is the only one showing any response to auditory input. Her parents will be investigating local rehabilitation services to provide individual therapy for speech and language skills and auditory training.

Should the readers have any questions or should additional information be needed, please feel free to contact me at XXX-XXXX.

Audiologist

CC:

Section V Other Physiological Assessments

Protocol 20 Facial Nerve Electroneurography

Target Population:
Patients who have suffered acute facial paralysis as a result of idiopathic (Bell's) palsy, trauma (including post surgical trauma) herpes zoster oticus, viral infections such as chicken pox and mumps, or otologic infections. In general, the evaluation should occur no sooner than 48-72 hours and no later than 21 days after paralysis onset. Evaluations too soon after onset will not show the full extent of damage and evaluations after 21 days have questionable prognostic value.

Rationale:
Facial nerve electroneurography (ENOG) attempts to determine the quantity of electrically stimulable nerve fibers remaining on the side of paralysis. This is done by comparing the amplitudes of the responses recorded from each side of the face.

Equipment Required:
Evoked potential system with somatosensory stimulation capability
Surface electrodes e.g., mini cup electrodes
Materials for applying electrodes
    alcohol swabs, abrasive solution (e.g. Nu-Prep™, OMNI-PREP ®), gauze pads, conductive cream (e.g., SYNAPSE®)
Somatosensory probe

Methods:
1.   Take a brief history and observe both sides of the face while the patient attempts to smile and close eyes. Classify the facial nerve dysfunction as a House-Brackmann (HB) Grade I-VI (refer to the reverse side of the ENOG Worksheet (Appendix B). Record the HB Grade, the suspected cause of the paralysis, date of onset, and the referring physician on the ENOG Worksheet (Appendix A).

2.   Electrode configuration: active: nasolabial fold test side
                                 reference: nasolabial fold opposite side
                                 ground: nape of neck

3.   Apply electrodes as follows:
    a.   clean skin with alcohol pad
    b.   using a gauze pad moistened with abrasive solution, rub skin until it is pink
    c.   place conductive cream in cup electrode and secure with clear adhesive tape
    Also, at the site of stimulation below each pinna, clean the skin and rub with abrasive solution.

4.   Plug the electrodes into the patient connection box and record impedances on the ENOG Worksheet. The impedances should be ≤ 3 kohm.

5.   Set up the acquisition parameters (Appendix C) and record on the ENOG Worksheet, maintaining a record of each trial.

6.   Place conductive cream on tips of somatosensory probe. Place one tip of the probe in the stylomastoid foramen just below the lobe of the pinna and the other tip slightly above and in front of the foramen, near the lobe of the pinna. Start with either side. If the patient is anxious, start with the paralyzed side as the stimulation is less noxious and it is the more important side to test. Obtaining a response from the normal side assures that the system is functioning properly. Adjust the current output to the about 15 mA. For young children or adults with slender necks, you may want to start with 10 mA on the normal side. When the desired current level is achieved, collect several sweeps for an average. Save and view the response. Blocking should be used to eliminate the artifact.

7.   Whether a response is present or not, increase the current in 5 mA steps, collecting averages at each level until either the peak - peak amplitude doesn't increase, the patient can't tolerate the stimulus, or the maximum current (40 mA) is reached. A good response has a positive-going peak at about 5 ms followed by a broader negative peak at about 10 ms (see Appendix D).

8.   Repeat steps 6 and 7 on the opposite side.

9.   To analyze the results, place one cursor on the positive peak and the other on the negative peak (or on the baseline of the tracing if no negative peak occurs) and record the peak-to-peak (or baseline-to-peak) amplitude of the largest response(s) on each side (see Appendix D). A good prognosis is noted if the response amplitude on the paralyzed side is at least 10% of the response amplitude on the normal side. A poor prognosis results if the amplitude on the paralyzed side is less than 10% of the amplitude on the normal side.

Report Format:
Patient identification (name and Hospital #), waveforms, and response amplitudes should be printed on the Auditory Brainstem Response Audiometry Form (see Appendix D). Waveforms should be labeled as to the side stimulated and the current level used. Any changes from standard protocol must also be recorded and any other information that may be useful in interpretation may be added.

A written report should be placed in the chart and sent to the referring doctor(see Appendix E).

Billing:
Bill Electroneurography (CPT 92516) in 15 minute units.

References:
Beck, D. L., & Benecke, J. E. (1993). Electroneurography: Electrical evaluation of the facial nerve. *Journal of the American Academy of Audiology, 4*, 109-115.

Beck, D. L. (1993). Facial nerve electrophysiology: Electroneurography and facial nerve monitoring. *Seminars in Hearing, 14*, 123-133.

Protocol 20 Appendix

ELECTRONEUROGRAPHY WORKSHEET

NAME: _____   HOSP. ID _____

BIRTHDATE _____-_____-_____   DATE _____-_____-_____

SUSPECTED CAUSE _____   DATE OF ONSET ___-___-___

HOUSE-BRACKMANN GRADE _____   REFERRING PHYSICIAN _____

ELECTRODE MONTAGE: ACTIVE ___   ELECTRODE IMPEDANCE

              REFERENCE ___

              GROUND ___

RECORD	SIDE	STIM LEVEL (mA)	PULSE DUR (μs)	STIM RATE (pps)	FILTERS	RESPONSE AMPLITUDE (μV)	COMMENTS
1			150	1	1-3000		
2							
3							
4							
5							
6							
7							
8							
9							
10							
11							
12							
13							
14							
15							
16							
17							
18							
19							

ELECTRONEUROGRAPHY WORKSHEET (REVERSE SIDE)

Facial Nerve Grading System

I	Normal	Normal facial function in all areas

II Mild dysfunction

Gross: slight weakness noticeable on close inspection; may have very slight synkinesis
At rest: normal symmetry and tone
Motion
Forehead: moderate to good function
Eye: complete closure with minimum effort
Mouth: slight asymmetry

III Moderate dysfunction

Gross: obvious but not disfiguring difference between two sides: noticeable but not severe synkinesis, contracture, and/or hemifacial spasm
At rest: normal symmetry and tone
Motion
Forehead: slight to moderate movement
Eye: complete closure with effort
Mouth: slightly weak with maximum effort

IV Moderately severe
       dysfunction

Gross: obvious weakness and/or disfiguring asymmetry
At rest: normal symmetry and tone
Motion
Forehead: none
Eye: incomplete closure

V Severe dysfunction

Gross: only barely perceptible motion
At rest: asymmetry
Motion
Forehead: none
Eye: incomplete closure
Mouth: slight movement

VI Total paralysis   No movement

From House J. W., & Brackmann E. D. (1985). Facial nerve grading system. *Otolaryngology Head Neck Surgery, 9,* 146.

MOUTH MOVEMENT	EYE CLOSURE	AT REST	HB GRADE
NORMAL	NORMAL	NORMAL	I
SLIGHT ASYMMETRY	COMPLETE W/MIN	NORMAL	II
WEAK W/ MAX EFFORT	EFFORT	NORMAL	III
WEAK W/ MAX EFFORT	COMPLETE W/ EFFORT	NORMAL	IV
SLIGHT MOVEMENT	INCOMPLETE	ASYMMETRY\	V
NONE	INCOMPLETE	LOSS OF TONE	VI
	NONE		

ELECTRONEUROGRAPHY SET-UP PARAMETERS

GENERAL SETUP   AMPLIFIER SETUP
                                          Channel 1
Test: ENOG   Gain: 1000
Channels: 1   Hi Filter: 3000
Window: 20.000   Low Filter: 3
Pre/Post: 0   Notch filter: out
Points: 256   Artifact: disabled
                                      Montage: nasolabial fold/nape
                                      Distance 0

                  STIMULUS SETUP
                  Stimulator: somato   probe   :unilateral #1
                  Max # Stim.: 256   duration   :150
                  Rate (/s): 1

EXAMPLE OF ELECTRONEUROGRAPHY WAVEFORM

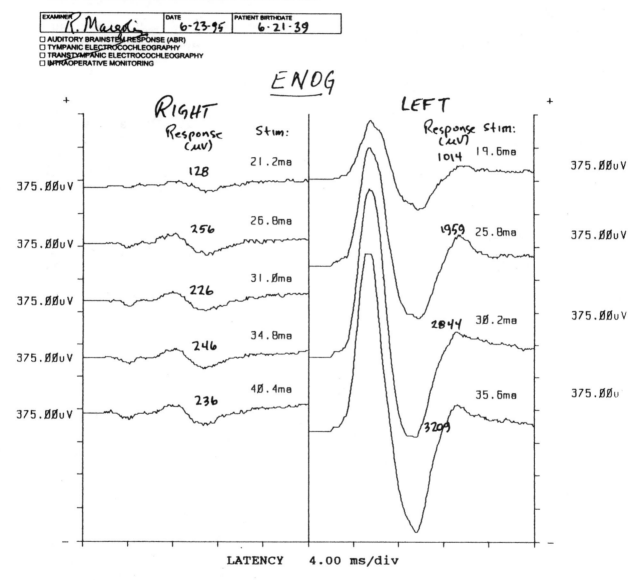

UNIVERSITY OF MINNESOTA HOSPITAL AND CLINIC
AUDIOLOGY CLINIC
AUDITORY EVOKED POTENTIALS

| EXAMINER R. Margoli | DATE 6-23-95 | PATIENT BIRTHDATE 6·21·39 |

☐ AUDITORY BRAINSTEM RESPONSE (ABR)
☐ TYMPANIC ELECTROCOCHLEOGRAPHY
☐ TRANSTYMPANIC ELECTROCOCHLEOGRAPHY
☐ INTRAOPERATIVE MONITORING

ENOG

RIGHT
Response (uV)   Stim:

LEFT
Response (uV)   Stim:

128	21.2ms
256	26.8ms
226	31.0ms
246	34.8ms
236	40.4ms

1014	19.6ms
1959	25.8ms
2844	30.2ms
3209	35.6ms

375.00uV
375.00uV
375.00uV
375.00uV
375.00uV

375.00uV
375.00uV
375.00uV
375.00u

+   +

LATENCY   4.00 ms/div

EXAMPLE OF ELECTRONEUROGRAPHY REPORT

Patient Name
Hospital ID #

BACKGROUND:
     The patient was referred by Dr. N for facial nerve electroneurography. He is four days out from an injury to the right side of the head. He appears to have a slight movement of the mouth and incomplete closure of the eye with maximal effort.

PROCEDURES AND RESULTS:
     Facial nerve function was assessed by stimulating the area of the stylomastoid foramen and recording the evoked EMG from the ipsilateral nasolabial fold. Reference and ground electrodes were placed on the contralateral nasolabial fold and neck, respectively.
     Responses were obtained from both sides of the face. (See the Auditory Evoked Potentials form.) The maximum response amplitude from the right side was about 7% of the maximum response from the left side. The response peaks on the right were also delayed compared to the left side.

INTERPRETATION:
     The results suggest poor facial nerve function on the right side. A response amplitude less than 10% of the response amplitude from the unaffected side suggests a poor prognosis for spontaneous recovery.

Audiologist

Protocol 21
Vestibular Function Tests:
Electronystagmography and Rotation

Target Population:
1.   Patients who have symptoms of vertigo, disequilibrium, or imbalance due to an underlying disease condition. This might involve the inner ear (Meniere's syndrome and labyrinthitis), the vestibular nerve (e.g. vestibular neuronitis and acoustic neuroma), cervical muscles and vertebrae (whiplash injuries), or the central nervous system (e.g. basilar artery migraine, demyelinating diseases such as multiple sclerosis, neurodegeneration such as hereditary ataxias, tumors, and infarcts).

2.   Patients who are receiving medications that might impair inner ear function. Ototoxic drugs include the aminoglycoside antibiotics (e.g., gentamicin) and some diuretics (e.g., furosemide) when they are used in conjunction with other ototoxic medications.

3.   Patients who are recovering from inner ear or vestibular nerve surgery and continue to have symptoms of vertigo or disequilibrium. The surgery might have been resection of an acoustic neuroma or a vestibular nerve section for intractable Meniere's disease.

Rationale:
The term electronystagmography has been used for the set of tests including the following: caloric stimulation; screening tests for saccades, pursuit eye tracking, and optokinetic stimulation; and evaluation of spontaneous eye movements during maintained head positions and the Hallpike maneuver. Tests using rotation of the subject, sometimes referred to as slow harmonic oscillation, are frequently done along with the calorics and will be included as part of the ENG test battery. The ENG and rotation test battery can identify a vestibular deficit affecting eye movements and the vestibulo-ocular reflex (VOR) and determine whether there is a bilateral deficit or an asymmetry due to decreased function (or increased) on one side compared to the other side. In addition, it is useful for determining whether there is an oculomotor deficit which might involve central nervous system pathways in common with the vestibular system. Dynamic posturography (Protocol 22) complements the ENG and provides information about whether there is a vestibular deficit affecting postural stability.

Equipment Required:
EOG electrodes (silver/silver chloride disks, 2-3 mm diameter) with shielded leads
Amplifiers for EOG electrodes
Computerized data acquisition and display system
Visual stimulus generator
Caloric irrigation unit

Computer driven rotation chair

Methods:

1.   Otoscopic inspection. Before caloric stimulation, the ear canals should be inspected for excessive cerumen and active ear disease. Excessive cerumen should be removed (Protocol 3). If there is evidence for ear disease, a physician should be consulted.

2.   Preparation of skin before electrode placement. The skin should be cleaned with an alcohol pad, using gentle rubbing to remove any oils on the surface of the skin.

3.   EOG electrodes. These record the corneoretinal potential, which is proportional to the position of the eye in the head (Young & Sheena, 1975). The electrodes are covered with an electrode cream to ensure a uniform electrical contact with the skin and placed on the surface of the skin: a) on the lateral canthi of each eye (for recording of horizontal eye movements) and b) above and below one eye to record the vertical movements of that eye. The electrodes should be pressed firmly against the skin and tape used to keep the electrode in contact with the skin. For grounding purposes, an electrode can be placed in the midline of the forehead or a metal plate can be placed on the wrist. It is important to minimize any artifacts due to movement of the electrode relative to the skin and any recording of EMG and EKG potentials.

4.   Adaptation to ambient light level. After the electrodes are taped to the skin, the patient should be placed in the testing room and the background light level in the room adjusted to that used for the first tests. No recording should be made for at least 5 minutes whenever there is a significant change in the background illumination, because the magnitude of the corneoretinal potential (which is recorded by the EOG electrodes) is dependent upon the amount of light or dark adaptation of the retina. If that changes, then the system would need to be recalibrated.

5.   Calibration of the EOG measurement system. The patient is seated in an exam chair with his/her head fixed with a head holder (to keep the head from moving) and instructed to look at a small red spot (either a marker or a projected spot of light; see 7 and 8 below) positioned on the wall or screen directly in front of the patient. The spot is positioned equally to the right and left of the midline(e.g., 20 degrees to either side) for calibrating the horizontal electrodes and above and below the midline for calibrating the vertical electrodes. While the patient is looking at the spot, the EOG signals and a signal proportional to the position of the light beam are sampled and stored in the computer. This is done at the beginning and end of each individual test in the ENG battery and also after any significant change in the background illumination. The actual calibration number (degrees per volt) is calculated as follows. The visual angle between the right and left (or top and bottom) target lights relative to the midpoint between the patient's eyes is calculated and that is divided by the difference in the voltage of the EOG electrodes when the patient was looking to the right and left (or top and bottom). The resulting number has units of degrees per volt, and the EOG signals must be multiplied by it. For any given test, the average of the calibrations obtained just before and after that test should be used.

6.   Optokinetic (OK) stimulation. After the patient is adapted to a dimly light room, the OK pattern is rotated in the horizontal plane. This is the optokinetic stimulus. There are several possibilities for generating the OK pattern: a) rotating a drum which surrounds the patient and has alternating black and white vertical strips (with a spatial frequency of 0.16 Hz) or has a random pattern of black spots on a white background, b) rotating a cylinder placed in front of the patient which has alternating black and white stripes, or c) moving a pattern across a computer display screen positioned in front of the patient. The "strongest" stimulus (i.e., the

one causing the greatest nystagmus) is rotation of a random dot pattern which surrounds the patient. Four rotations of the visual pattern are used: rotations with a constant velocity of 45 deg/s and 90 deg/s, to the right and left. The velocity of the slow phases of the nystagmus is quantified.

7.   Horizontal pursuit eye tracking. A spot of light (0.5 deg. in diameter) is rear projected onto a screen, 60 inches in front of the patient's eyes. The light spot is created by a laser beam which is reflected off two servo controlled galvanometer mirrors. The position of the mirrors is controlled by a voltage that can be generated with a stand alone function generator or by means of the digital to analog output of the computer's data acquisition card. It is moved sinusoidally in the horizontal direction at 0.2 Hz, with a peak displacement of 20 deg. to either side of the midline. Two parameters are calculated: a) the percentage of the eye movement that is saccadic and b) the maximum velocity of the smooth component of the eye movement.

8.   Saccadic eye movements. The target light (same as for the pursuit task) is displayed directly in front of the patient and 20 deg. to either side. The light is moved suddenly (within 3 ms) from one position to the next after a random delay of 1 to 3 s. Note: If a laser light system is not available, then the patient can look at discreet spots on the screen (or wall), positioned 20 deg. to the right and left of midline. This can also be used for calibrating the EOG electrodes. The latency, peak velocity, and amplitude of the eye movement are calculated.

9.   Maintained head position. The subject is seated upright in a chair that has a reclining back. The patient sits quietly for five minutes in a darkened room or with light-tight goggles over the eyes for at least five minutes (for dark adaptation of the retina which will stabilize the baseline of the EOG signal). Four trials (45 s each) are recorded under the following conditions: a) The patient is seated in the upright position. b) The back of the chair is tilted backward so that the patient is lying with the head supine (looking to the ceiling). c) The head is slowly turned 45 deg to one side and then held there for the recording. d) The head is slowly turned to the other side and held there.   If a sustained nystagmus is present, the velocity of the slow phases is calculated.

10.   Hallpike maneuver. The subject is seated upright on the exam chair with the head rest removed and with the back tilted backward. The examiner carefully but firmly holds the patient's head. The head is rapidly positioned backward and turned to one side, in one continuous movement so that the posterior semicircular on that side is excited. When there is no longer any nystagmus, then the patient is slowly brought back to the upright position. This procedure is repeated with the head turned to the other side. Under visual inspection by the examiner and with the EOG recording, the direction (horizontal, vertical, or rotatory), latency, and duration of any nystagmus are determined. If there is a nystagmus, then the maneuver is repeated to see if the nystagmus response fatigues, i.e., diminishes on subsequent trials.

11.   Rotation of the subject in complete darkness. The patient is placed in the rotation chair, the safety harnesses and seat belt are fastened, and the head is secured to a holder and positioned so that the horizontal semicircular canals are approximately in the horizontal plane. If there was any change in the ambient light level during or after the position tests, then the patient sits quietly for dark adaptation. Thereafter, a calibration recording is made, and then the patient is rotated in complete darkness or with goggles so that there is no visual stimulation. Rotation is in the horizontal plane and stimulates the horizontal semicircular canal afferents. Two types of rotation are used: a) Constant acceleration in one direction. The patient is first rotated at a

constant velocity of 90 deg/s. After the nystagmus (due to the acceleration from no rotation to 90 deg/s) has ceased, a baseline condition is established. The stimulus conditions are:

      a.   A period of constant acceleration (18 s at 10 deg/s^2 acceleration and 9 s at 20 deg/s^2 acceleration) which causes the chair to smoothly slow down and then change direction until it rotates at 90 deg/s in the opposite direction. There are four trials (two different magnitudes of acceleration in both directions, right and left). The recording for each trial starts 5 s before the acceleration begins and continues until the nystagmus is gone. The maximum and the time constant for the velocity of the slow phases of the nystagmus are calculated.

      b.   Sinusoidal rotation. The frequencies are 0.05, 0.1, 0.5, and 1 Hz. The peak chair velocity is 60 deg/s up to 0.5 Hz and 30 deg/s at 1.0 Hz. The actual velocity of the chair is sampled along with the EOG signals. The phase and gain of the slow phase of the nystagmus, relative to the chair velocity, are calculated.

12.   <u>Caloric stimulation.</u> The patient lies backward in the examination chair and with the head tilted backward about 60 deg. (relative to the normal horizontal position) so that the horizontal semicircular canals are approximately in the vertical plane. Two different stimuli, warm air and ice water, are used for each ear. The EOG recording starts when the stimulus begins and continues until the nystagmus is gone.

      a.   Warm air: 50 deg C is applied to the external ear canal for 90 s (with a constant flow of 7-11 l/min).

      b.   Ice water: 30 cc are applied (with a syringe cooled in the ice water) to the external ear canal over 15-20 s.

13.   <u>Visual suppression of a vestibular nystagmus.</u> The patient is asked to fixate on a spot of light straight ahead in from of the face during vestibular stimulation. This can be done during caloric stimulation, but preferably during the rotation tests. For the latter, the following can be used: a) sinusoidal rotation at 0.2 Hz, or b) constant acceleration at 10 deg/s^2 (see 11 above). The percent reduction in the eye velocity is quantified. Abnormal suppression (i.e. not enough reduction in the vestibular nystagmus) indicates CNS (brainstem/cerebellar) dysfunction.

14.   <u>Interpretation.</u> An asymmetry of greater than 25% for the calorics or rotation is significant. If the maximum eye velocity is not greater than normal (i.e., not "hyperactive"), then this indicates a unilateral weakness or deficit. Dysmetric saccades (over or undershoot of the target) or abnormal use of saccades during pursuit tracking indicate CNS dysfunction, possibly involving the brainstem and cerebellum.

Report Format:

The EOG and stimulus waveforms are sampled and saved on a computer disk. The data are analyzed off-line. One of the laboratory personnel first reviews all of the recordings on a computer monitor in order to identify any artifacts. The data are then analyzed and the parameter values inserted into a formatted spreadsheet file. Finally, the Summary and the Conclusion are completed by entering text into designated sections of the spreadsheet file. This serves as a concise summary report and copies are inserted into the patient's hospital chart. An example of a summary report in included in Appendix A. Graphs of the actual eye movement recordings for the ENG and rotation tests and the sway and strategy scores for posturography (See Protocol 22) can also be inserted into the chart, depending on the needs of the referring physician.

Billing:

Standard CPT codes are used for submitting requests for reimbursement. The codes are used for the performance of the tests, and analysis and interpretation of the results with no time constraints. The following codes can be used for the standard tests.

92270	Eye Saccade-Horizontal
92541	Spontaneous Nystagmus
92542	Positional Nystagmus
92543	Calorics: bilateral
92544	Optokinetic Stimulation
92545	Oscillatory Tracking
92546	Rotation
92547	Vertical Recording
92567	Impedance Fistula

References:

Baloh, R. W., Sills, A. W., & Honrubia, V. (1979). Impulsive and sinusoidal rotatory testing: A comparison with results of caloric testing. *Laryngoscope, 89,* 646-654.

Cyr, D. G. (1991). Vestibular system assessment. In Rintelmann, W.F. (Ed.) *Hearing Assessment.* Austin, TX: Pro-Ed, pp. 739-804.

Demer, J. L. (1995). Evaluation of vestibular and visual oculomotor function. *Otolaryngology, Head and Neck Surgery, 112,* 16-35.

Honrubia, V. (1995). Contemporary vestibular function testing: Accomplishments and future perspectives. *Otolaryngology, Head and Neck Surgery, 112,* 64-77.

Houston, H. G., & Watson, D. R. (1994). A review of computerized electronystagmography technology. *British Journal of Audiology, 28,* 41-46

Scherer, H., Teiwes, W., & Clark, A. H. (1991). Measuring three dimensions of eye movement in dynamic situations by means of video-oculography. *Acta Otolaryngologica, 111,* 182-187.

Young, L. R., & Sheena, D. (1975). Eye movement measurement techniques. *American Psychologist, 30,* 315-330.

Protocol 21 Appendix

A.   Example of Vestibular Report

EXAMPLE OF VESTIBULAR REPORT

Birth Date:

Age: Sex:

Referred By:

Hosp ID:
Name:
Lab ID:

Test Date:

HISTORY

Vertigo: Has been having episodes of nystagmus. 1st episode occurred in early 1993. The nystagmus was witnessed by a number of people at his office. This episode lasted the longest, about 2 minutes. He has been doing fairly well recently, but in May he had fairly frequent minor episodes that lasted 10-20 seconds. The nystagmus usually occurs when he's moving, but once occurred when sitting at a theater.

Hearing: High frequency loss bilaterally due to noise exposure in the past.

Tinnitus: Constant bilateral ringing, louder on the R than the L

REFER DIAG: CNS vs. peripheral vestibular dysfunction.

TESTS PERFORMED

ROTATION: Deg/s²

	10	20			
R accel:	-10	-13			
L accel:	2	2			
Asymmetry:	-83%	-87%			

CALORICS:

	Cold:Vel	Dur	Warm:Vel	Dur		Aysmm	Prepond
R stim:	0		-1				
L stim:	-2		-1			-7%	

POSITION: Maintained head position in the dark: strong nystagmus, slow phase to R; supine : ~ 7 deg/s.

HALLPIKE: No dizziness.

GAZE: Hor.: square wave jerks in the light; higher frequency in the dark.

PURSUIT: Vert.: normal up; borderline saccadic down.

Hor.: mildly saccadic to R

SACCADES: Vert. & hor: normal amplitude.

POSTURE: Sensory: (1) Sway-referenced gain = 1.0: fell on conditions 5, 6; normal for other conditions.

(2) Reduced sway-ref. gain = 0.5 ("easier"):borderline low for c 5, 6.

Motor: (1) Forward translation of platform: normal strength & latency.

(2) Back translation of plat.: normal strength & latency

EXAMPLE OF VESTIBULAR REPORT *page 2*

SUMMARY:

*   1. Calorics: no definite response for either ear.

*   2. Rotation of subject in complete darkness: a) definite response for rotation to the R at 10 deg/s^2; b) during sinusoidal rotation, definite responses during rotation in both directions; same max in both directions after subtracting for spontan.

*   3. Spontaneous nystagmus in the dark: slow phase to R.

*   4. Square wave jerks in light & darkness.

*   5. Pursuit eye tracking (horizontal): saccadic.

*   6. Posturography: a) sensory: fell for conditions 5 and 6.

CONCLUSION:

1. Profound bilateral vestibular deficit, but some function present (based on constant acceleration and sinusoidal rotation).

2. Definite oculomotor abnormalities.

3. Both the VOR and postural stability were severely affected by the bilateral vestibular deficit.

4. Vestibular & oculomotor dysfunction due to cerebellar/brainstem dysfunction.

Protocol 22
Vestibular Function Tests:
Dynamic Posturography (DP)

Target Population:
1. Patients complaining of vertigo, disequilibrium, or imbalance.

2. Patients who are being followed to determine whether there is progression of a disease state that affects the balance mechanisms (as in some hereditary ataxias) or to differentiate among several subtypes of the disease condition.

3. Patients undergoing balance training or physical therapy. DP can help to develop a plan that takes into account the specific problems of an individual patient.

4. Patients with a history of falls and elderly patients with a sense of disequilibrium.

5. Patients who are being evaluated for balance problems after head trauma.

Rationale:
The term posturography refers to the quantitative measurement of body sway or center of force exerted at the feet while the patient stands on a platform. Dynamic refers to measurements taken while the platform is moving as well as when it is stationary. Only body movement in the forward/backward plane will be considered. Since DP evaluates the vestibulo-spinal system and the function of the vertical semicircular canals and otolith organs, it complements the ENG and rotation tests. There might be an abnormality in one or more of the different components of the vestibular system, and DP can thus help to provide a more comprehensive evaluation of the patient's problem.

Dynamic posturography provides unique information that can help to identify whether postural instability is due to a deficit in or inability to use sensory information from the inner ear, eye, or the cutaneous receptors of the feet and the proprioceptors of the joints and muscles of the leg, or to a combination of the different sensory modalities. There might be a pattern of responses across the different DP test conditions that would suggest a specific disease condition. However, DP itself (with the standard Equitest™ protocol) does not provide site of lesion, or laterality information.

Equipment Required:
Equitest™ platform with visual surround

Computerized data acquisition and display system that is integrated with the platform controller and force transducers
Safety harness

Methods:

1. _Tests._ The protocol uses two sets of test conditions, designated as sensory organization and motor control. However, only the sensory organization tests were designed for evaluating the vestibular system, and the motor control tests will not be described here. For each condition, the computer samples five force transducers mounted under the platform: four that measure the vertical thrust on the platform and one that measures the horizontal shear force. From these measurements, several parameters are computed.

For the sensory organization tests, six different conditions are used. For each condition, there are three trials, each lasting 20 s. The conditions are:
   1.   Stable platform. Eyes open and stationary visual surround.
   2.   Stable platform. Eyes closed.
   3.   Stable platform. Eyes open with a moving visual surround.
   4.   Moving platform. Eyes open and stationary visual surround.
   5.   Moving platform. Eyes closed.
   6.   Moving platform. Eyes open with a moving visual surround.
There are two parameters that are calculated. a) Equilibrium score. The center of force is calculated and used to estimate the peak-to-peak change in forward/backward body sway. This is expressed as an equilibrium score. A score of 100 indicates no sway and a score of 0 indicates that the patient fell into the harness. b) Strategy score. This is the peak-to-peak change in the shear force, divided by 25 lbs. This score has been interpreted as indicating the relative amount of hip vs. ankle movement, although biomechanical modeling studies indicate that this is not always the case (Barin, 1989). The equilibrium scores are more easily interpreted and have been the most useful.

2.   Interpretation. Under conditions five and six, the patient must rely on the vestibular inputs for maintaining balance. There is no vision (eyes closed) and the platform is moving, which reduces the inputs from the joint receptors of the ankle and muscle receptors of the lower leg muscles. Abnormally low scores on 5 and 6, but normal on the other conditions, indicates a significant vestibular deficit. It could be bilateral or an uncompensated unilateral deficit. Other patterns of sway across the different sensory conditions have been reported and are still under investigation (Furman, 1994).

Billing:
Bill CPT code 92599 for dynamic posturography.

Report Format:
Results of Dynamic Posturography are summarized and interpretation included in the vestibular report (See Protocol 21, Appendix A). Graphs of sway and strategy scores and raw movement can be included with the vestibular report (see Appendix A).

References:

Barin, K. (1992). Dynamic posturography. Analysis of error in force plate measurement of postural sway. *IEEE Engineering in Medicine and Biology, 11,* 52-56.

Cyr, D. G. (1991). Vestibular system assessment. In Rintelmann, W.F. (Ed.) *Hearing Assessment.* Austin, TX: Pro-Ed, pp. 739-804.

Furman, J. (1995). Role of posturography in management of vestibular patients. *Otolaryngology, Head and Neck Surgery, 112,* 8-15.

Nashner, L. M., Black F. O., & Wall, C. (1982). Adaptation to altered support and visual conditions during stance: Patients with vestibular deficits. *Journal of Neuroscience, 2,* 536-544.

Protocol 22 Appendix

A.   **Equitest Summary**

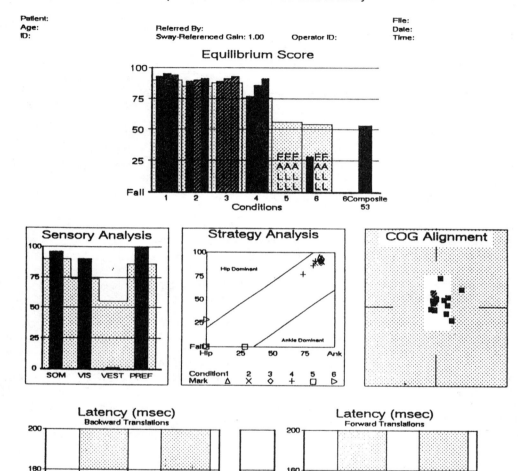

EQUITEST SUMMARY
Equilibrium & Balance Laboratory

Patient:
Age:
ID:

Referred By:
Sway-Referenced Gain: 1.00   Operator ID:

File:
Date:
Time:

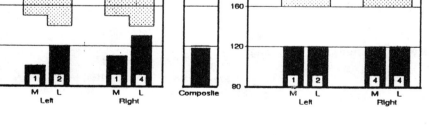

Index